Medicine In The Bible

John Yeung

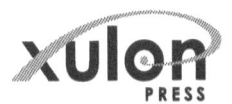

Copyright © 2003 by John Yeung

Medicine In The Bible
by John Yeung

Printed in the United States of America

Library of Congress Control Number: 2003102308
ISBN 1-591606-35-7

All rights reserved. No part of this publication may be reproduced or transmitted in any form or by any means without written permission of the publisher.

Unless otherwise indicated, Bible quotations are taken from the New International Version © Copyright 1973, 1978, 1984 by International Bible Society, or the New King James Version © Copyright 1979, 1980, 1982, 1984 by Thomas Nelson Publishers.

Xulon Press
www.xulonpress.com

To order additional copies, call 1-866-909-BOOK (2665).

Table of Contents

Preface ix

Foreword xv

The Five-Year Training of Medical Students in Universities and Hospitals Is Approximately as Follows:

YEAR 1 & 2: Study of Anatomy, Physiology, Biochemistry, Medical Sciences, Genetics

Chapter 1	Why Were the Hairs of Absalom so Heavy? (Physiology)...17
Chapter 2	Why Did King David Need a Girl to Treat His Coldness? (Biochemistry) 23
Chapter 3	The Principle to Explain Revelation (Anatomy)..29
Chapter 4	How Could Jesus Become Bright During the Transfiguration? (Genetics) 35
Chapter 5	The Experiment by Noah (Epidemiology) 39

YEAR 3: Study of Pathology, Forensic Medicine, Pharmacology, Microbiology

Chapter 6	What is the Purpose of Sour Wine in Crucifixion? (Pharmacology).....................45
Chapter 7	The Death of Jesus (Pathology) 53

Chapter 8	The Ten Plagues and Microorganisms (Microbiology)	61
Chapter 9	How Did Cain Kill Abel? (Forensic Medicine)	71

Interlude 75

YEAR 4: Study of Medicine, Emergency Medicine, Sports Medicine, Anesthesia, Surgery

Chapter 10	Sleeping Disorders of Samson, David and Jesus (Medicine: Neurology)	87
Chapter 11	Sexually Transmitted Diseases (STDs) and Repentance (Medicine)	95
Chapter 12	Running and the Advice of Paul (Sports Medicine)	101
Chapter 13	Emergency of Lazarus and the Timing of Jesus (Emergency Medicine)	105
Chapter 14	Did Adam Have One Rib Less than Eve? (Anesthesia)	113
Chapter 15	Circumcision and the Intelligence of God (Surgery)	119
Chapter 16	The Demon-Possessed Man in Garasenes (Surgery: Transplantation)	125

YEAR 5: Study of Obstetrics, Gynecology, Orthopedics, Pediatrics, Radiology, Oncology, Ear, Nose & Throat (ENT), Ophthalmology, Psychiatry

Chapter 17	No Let-up in Heavy Menstrual Bleeding (Gynecology)	131
Chapter 18	The Pregnancies of Sarah and Rebekah (Obstetrics)	135

Table of Contents

Chapter 19	Bones and Pop Music (Orthopedics)	141
Chapter 20	How Could Nicodemus Be Born Again? (Pediatrics)	145
Chapter 21	The Healing of Blindness (Ophthalmology)	151
Chapter 22	Hear the End of Age (ENT)	161
Chapter 23	The Law Concerning Our Teeth (Dentistry)	169
Chapter 24	X-rays and the Judgment of Jesus (Radiology)	179
Chapter 25	Similarity Between Sin and Cancer (Oncology)	185
Chapter 26	Did Jesus Have Anxiety? (Psychiatry)	191

At last 197
Author's Biography...199
Book Summary 201

Preface

Do you think that the Bible is just a book of history?

Do you believe that our knowledge today can be found in the Bible?

Do you believe that our knowledge today can help to account for some facts in the Bible?

If you find any knowledge in the Bible and want to share it, may I encourage you here to join me in writing a series of architecture in the Bible, law in the Bible, science in the Bible, art in the Bible, economics in the Bible, mathematics in the Bible, music in the Bible, history in the Bible, business in the Bible, etc.

Please let me know if you will join me.

May the Lord unveil His face and update His words for us.

Suggestion for Reading This Book

Please do not skip the scriptures quoted although sometimes they may be long. You might be very familiar with those verses in the Bible but please read them carefully once more.

Notice

Medicine is an ever-changing science. As new research and clinical experience broaden our knowledge, changes in treatment and drug therapy are required. The author has checked with sources believed to be reliable in his effort to provide information that is concise and generally in accord with the standards accepted at the time of publication. However, in view of the possibility of changes in medical sciences or human error, neither the author nor the publisher nor any other party who has been involved in the preparation or publication of this work warrants that the information contained herein is in every respect accurate or complete, and they disclaim all responsibility for any errors or omissions or for the results obtained from use of the information contained in this work. Readers are encouraged to confirm the information contained herein with other sources. Some information was simplified in order to make this book easy to read. For example, 37.1 million became 37 million; hepatitis B infection can cause liver cancer, liver failure and cirrhosis but only liver cancer was mentioned.

Foreword

In the beginning of writing this book, I thought I knew something and I decided to write and teach, to teach what I have known.

As I continued to write, I discovered that I knew little and I decided to write and share, to share what I might know.

Now, I am still writing but I really discover that I know nothing so I decide to write and learn, hoping someone can correct me after reading this book.

John Yeung
2002

Chapter 1

Why Were the Hairs of Absalom So Heavy? (Physiology)

What Is Physiology

Physiology is a fundamental science in medicine. It is the study of body functions. For instance, how a muscle contracts, how the kidney excretes urine, how nerves transmit impulses, how the lungs perform gaseous exchange, and how the hairs grow, etc. It is not difficult to think that a doctor has to know what is normal before he or she can diagnose the abnormal and treat it.

The Growth Of Our Hairs

Do you know how many hairs do we have? How long can it be if we don't have our hair cut for one year? Is there any medical significance by examining hairs?

In Matthew 10: 28–31

Jesus said, "Do not be afraid of those who kill the body but cannot kill the soul. Rather, be afraid of the One who can destroy both soul and body in hell. Are not two sparrows sold for a penny? Yet not one of them will fall to the ground apart from the will of your Father. And even the very hairs of your head are all numbered. So don't be afraid; you are worth more than many sparrows."

Jesus told us that God has numbered our hairs. Is it real? How many of them are there?

Approximately, our scalp has 100,000 hairs, eighty to ninety percent are in active growing (anagen) phase while ten percent are in resting (telogen) phase. Hairs are usually lost during the resting phase and about 100 hairs will be lost per day. Women in their pregnancy will have less hair lost but it will increase after childbirth[3]. The number of hair falling will be increased if one is sick.

In the above saying by Jesus, he told us that two sparrows sold for a copper coin and not one of them will fall if the Lord does not allow. So, what is the relationship between the falling of sparrows and the falling of our hairs? Can the falling of just two hairs from us be valuable too, let's say more expensive than a copper? If it is not, why bother God to count?

In fact, people will only do things when it can make profit. One will definitely count the number of sparrows falling as it is related to money: Two sparrows sold for a copper coin. Therefore four sparrows sold for two copper coins, six for three and so on. How can we increase the number of sparrows falling so that we can make more profit? Falling hairs in the ground is rubbish. People will remove it quickly together with the dust around it. No one will count that fall carefully unless they were made of gold. The only thing you will get by counting one's hairs and the number of hair falling is the person's health status. God cares for us and tries His best to gather our information in order to know us better. He counts our number of hairs and the hair falling every day. It is not because of money but love. Like the sparrows, not one of our hairs will fall to the ground apart from the will of our Father. (Note: The hair of famous people can now make profit as it can produce a clone).

Why Were Absalom's Hairs So Heavy

In 2 Samuel 14: 25–26

In all Israel there was not a man so highly praised for his handsome appearance as Absalom. From the top of his head to the sole of his foot there was no blemish in him. Whenever he cut the **hair** of his head — he used to cut his hair from time to time when it became too heavy for him — he would weigh it, and its weight was two hundred shekels by the royal standard.

The growth rate of hairs depends on numerous factors including our age, nutritional status, existing diseases, etc. Approximately, a hair will lengthen one mm in four days. Therefore the hairs will be about 9 cm longer if one does not have his hair cut for one year [3].

The weight of Absalom's hairs was 200 shekels (about 2.3 kg) when he had his hair cut each year. Can you guess what would happen if he did not have his hair cut for one or two years?

Probably, his head would be 4.6 kg heavier if he did not have his hair cut for just two years! The weight of hairs might pull his scalp with increasing discomfort. He might get headache easily whenever he moved his head vigorously, such as riding on a horse, playing wrestling game. So he might have his hair cut frequently in order to avoid such discomfort. But again, what made the hairs of Absalom so heavy?

Today, scientists use the heavy metal levels of human

hairs to determine the environmental exposure of mercury, arsenic, cadmium and lead as we know that excessive heavy metals exposure can lead to toxicity. High level of mercury in hairs may be the result of eating fish, especially big fish [1]. As big animals eat small animals, the resultant accumulation of heavy metals in big animals is therefore greater. High levels of arsenic, cadmium and lead may be the results of environmental exposure. It was found that children who eat dirt or clay and spend more time outdoors had higher hair heavy metal levels [2].

It may be very interesting to note that only the hairs of Absalom were that heavy compared to the other sons of David and the Israelites. In the Bible, there was no report of similar heavy hairs in the surrounding areas of Absalom. It therefore might not be a result of environmental exposure, otherwise some other people or his relatives might experience similar heavy hairs. It might be the result of his special habit. Perhaps he liked to eat big fish or other big animals from a source or a place which was heavily contaminated with heavy metals. If the place or source was in Israel, he might have consumed a large amount of such food compared to others. Therefore, it might be more reasonable to think that the place might have been far away from Israel if he was the only one to have such heavy hairs in the whole Israel. In fact, it was not difficult for a prince to get the food he wanted from other places.

Absalom was unique in the whole Israel. He was beautiful and his hair was heavy. He might be like a superstar that most people liked to mention him in their conversation. However, his heavy and beautiful hair did not bring him blessings; instead it was a leading cause of his death.

The Death of Absalom

Now Absalom happened to meet David's men. He

was riding his mule, and as the mule went under the thick branches of a large oak, Absalom's head got caught in the tree. He was left **hanging in midair**, while the mule he was riding kept on going. When one of the men saw this, he told Joab, "I just saw Absalom hanging in an oak tree."

Joab said to the man who had told him this, "What! You saw him? Why didn't you strike him to the ground right there? Then I would have had to give you ten shekels of silver and a warrior's belt."

But the man replied, "Even if a thousand shekels were weighed out into my hands, I would not lift my hand against the king's son. In our hearing the king commanded you and Abishai and Ittai, 'Protect the young man Absalom for my sake.' And if I had put my life in jeopardy and nothing is hidden from the king— you would have kept your distance from me."

Joab said, "I'm not going to wait like this for you." So he took three javelins in his hand and plunged them into Absalom's heart while Absalom was still alive in the oak tree. And ten of Joab's armor-bearers surrounded Absalom, struck him and killed him. (2 Samuel 18: 9–15)

References:

1. Centers for Disease Control and Prevention (CDC), "Blood and hair mercury levels in young children and women of childbearing age–United States, 1999," *MMWR Morbidity & Mortality Weekly Report* (2001): 50 (8): 140–3.
2. Hartwell, T.D., Handy, R.W., Harris, B.S., Williams, S.R., Gehlbach, S.H., "Heavy metal exposure in populations living around zinc and copper smelters," *Arch*

Environ Health, (1983): 38 (5): 284–95.
3. Shellow, W.V.R., "Approach to the patient with hair loss." In: Goroll, A.H., May, L.A., Mulley, A.G., "Primary care medicine: office evaluation and management of the adult patient," 4th ed. (Philadelphia: Lippincott Williams & Wilkins, 2000).

Chapter 2

Why Did King David Need a Girl to Treat His Coldness? (Biochemistry)

What Is Biochemistry

Most of us know what biochemistry is. For simplicity, it is the study of the chemical substances and vital processes occurring in living organisms, especially those inside humans.

In our secondary schools, we were taught what chemistry is — organic and inorganic. Most of the students (like me) feel bored when told to memorize those molecular formula, molecular weight and their reactions. Organic chemistry is the study of substances containing carbon, like starch, glucose, alcohol, proteins, fatty acids, etc. Inorganic chemistry therefore is the study of substances apart from organic matters, such as metals, chlorine. Biochemistry is something about the chemistry in the biological system, how energy is derived from food, how proteins are built and how DNAs and RNAs are formed, etc.

How can we get energy from food? Most of the energy is derived from complete breakdown of simple sugars through the Tricarboxylic acid (TCA) cycle [1]. The final products are water, carbon dioxide, energy in terms of adenosine triphosphate (ATP) molecules and heat. Even when we relax ourselves as far as we can, our muscles will not completely relax. There are still some contractions called muscle tone within some muscle fibers so that heat and our body temperature can therefore be produced. Only when we die will all of our muscles completely relax.

Why Did King David Feel Cold When He Was Old

In 1 Kings: 1–4

When King David was old and well advanced in years, he could **not** keep **warm** even when they put covers over him. So his servants said to him, "Let us look for a young virgin to attend the king and take care of him. She can lie beside him so that our lord, the king, may keep warm."
Then they searched throughout Israel for a beautiful girl and found Ab'ishag, a Shu'nammite, and brought her to the king. The girl was very beautiful; she took care of the king and waited on him, but the king had no intimate relations with her.

When King David became old, his muscle mass decreased and so did his metabolic rate. He could not generate enough heat and therefore felt cold all the day. He must have tried to put covers on him, such as the most expensive animal skins, and handmade clothes however he still felt cold. Nowadays we have different kinds of heating machines, oil based or heating wired types. If we cannot afford those expensive machines, we can simply buy some plastic heat packs which can we fill with hot water. (Note: Plastic is a polymer invented in the nineteenth century.) In the days of King David, there was no heating machine or heat pack no matter how rich you were.

Why Did King David Need a Girl to Treat His Coldness?

A Young Girl For Warming

Why did the servant of the King David bring him a girl for warming?

When I was a student, I usually got the hot water heat pack to warm myself in the winter night. However, it might be difficult to get an ideal temperature during sleeping. Sometimes it was too hot and sometimes it was too cold. The most troublesome was that it could only heat a small part of you. Usually our feet have the privilege to touch the heat pack as they are often the coldest part of the body. Later when I brought a heating machine, the room became a bit warmer but the air was too dry. My lips cracked and my throat felt sore. Some classmates suggested to place some glasses of water to increase the humidity but it obviously did not help much. Heating machine might be better when comparing heat pack except in the end of each month. The electric bill usually made me chill as it was always expensive. After I got married, I realized that humans are the best heating machines. One cold winter day, I worked late at night and went to bed immediately after finishing my work. I discovered that the bed was so warm to sleep. It was because my wife had already been in bed for hours. Her body temperature warmed the bed with the most optimal temperature, not too cold nor too hot (unless she is sick). The surface area that was covered was also optimal. It was also free. That was the time I realized why the servants of King David put a young girl beside him. Apart from warming, I think she could also be a spy, too.

Why Did Moses Not Feel Cold As David Did When He Was Old

In Deuteronomy 34: 1–12 (The Death of Moses)

Moses climbed Mount Nebo from the plains of Moab to the top of Pisgah, across from Jericho. There the Lord showed him the whole land — from Gilead to Dan, all of Naphtali, the territory of Ephraim and Manasseh, all the land of Judah as far as the western sea, the Negev and the whole region from the Valley of Jericho, the City of Palms, as far as Zoar. Then the Lord said to him, "This is the land I promised on oath to Abraham, Isaac and Jacob when I said, 'I will give it to your descendants.' I have let you see it with your eyes, but you will not cross over into it."

And Moses the servant of the Lord died there in Moab, as the Lord had said. **He buried him** in Moab, in the valley opposite Beth-peor, but to this day no one knows where his grave is. Moses was a hundred and twenty years old when he died, yet his eyes were not weak nor his strength gone. The Israelites grieved for Moses in the plains of Moab thirty days, until the time of weeping and mourning was over . . .

Since then, no prophet has risen in Israel like Moses, whom the Lord knew face-to-face, who did all those miraculous signs and wonders the Lord sent him to do in Egypt, to Pharaoh and to all his officials and to his whole land. For no one has ever shown the mighty power or performed the awesome deeds that Moses did in the sight of all Israel.

On the contrary, Moses, although in his age of one hundred and twenty, was still strong in body and faith. He seemed to be older than King David but appeared stronger. Although he spent most of his time in the desert where it should be colder, he was still healthier in his old age. Why? Can we compare the lifestyle of both leaders to find some clues of their health?

Moses, a servant of the Lord, indeed shared many similarities with King David. They both have killed and sinned. They both have been punished by God. They were both leaders of Israelites. They have written many chapters in the Bible.

There was however something different between them. Moses, whom the Lord knew face-by-face, performed all great terror and mighty power in the sight of Israel. King David, although a king, seldom did miraculous signs before Israel except casting out demon from Saul and winning battles.

God Is A Consuming Fire

In Deuteronomy 4: 21–24

Moses said, "The Lord was angry with me because of you, and he solemnly swore that I would not cross the Jordan and enter the good land the Lord your God is giving you as your inheritance. I will die in this land; I will not cross the Jordan; but you are about to cross over and take possession of that good land. Be careful not to forget the covenant of the Lord your God that he made with you; do not make for yourselves an idol in the form of anything the Lord your God has forbidden. For the Lord your God is a **consuming fire**, a jealous God."

In fact, it may be difficult to think why Moses was healthier than King David in their old age by just comparing their lifestyles. However, we may guess according to our limited knowledge that there may be an association between the exposure time of God's power and the underlying reason. Moses spent the second half of his life with the Lord after he met Him. King David, however, seemed to have left the Lord for an unknown period of time after he slept late till evening and knew Bathsheba, and killed her husband (a loyal servant of King David). God is a consuming fire. The face and body of Moses has been shown in the presence of God in the desert but the face of God had turned away for some time after David sinned. Without the presence of that consuming fire for some time when David was young, he therefore felt cold in his old age.

No one wants to become weak when he is old. All of us want to be forever green. Scientists do numerous researches to explore the method of being young and healthy. But what is the most effective and affordable method to be young and healthy?

References:

1. Brownie, A.C., Kernohan, J.C., Churchill's Mastery of Medicine: Biochemistry (Edinburgh: Churchill Livingstone, 1999).

Chapter 3

The Principle to Explain Revelation (Anatomy)

What Is Anatomy

Anatomy is the study of human structure, the positions of the organs, tissues and cells as well as their morphology. It is the science of the shape and structure of all organisms and its branches include embryology (study of fetal growth from fertilization till birth), gross anatomy (study of human with or without dissection under the naked eye), histology (study of human under light and electronic microscope), neuroanatomy (study of the anatomy of nervous tissues), etc.

All parts of our body have already been dissected and examined but not all dissection and examination yields knowledge. The brain may be the best example to verify this statement. Although the brain has been dissected, examined and named in very full details, most parts of it remain a mystery.

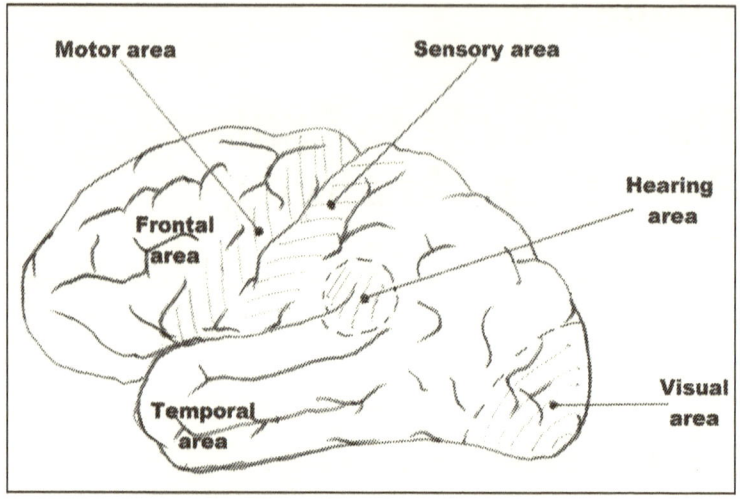

Figure 3.1 Different functions of the brain

It is just like Revelation in the Bible. Although we know every single word in it, we still do not know the meaning.

How To Explain Revelation

If a man suffers from frontal brain damage, he may have poor attention, and is easily distracted. He cannot memorize or is unable to form new memories, with a tendency to repeat words, phrases and actions. He may not be able to make plans and pursue goals, to deduce and generalize. His overall personality may change but there is no insight [1].

So, what is the exact function of the frontal brain according to the above description?

In fact, after detailed scientific observations about the consequences of the forebrain damage, the exact function remains obscure. We can only say that it is related to the higher functions of the brain such as personality, higher or abstract thinking, and so on.

How can we know the exact functions of different parts of

the brain and how can we know the meaning of Revelation?

To know the functions of the brain, we may do experiments according to what we observe. For example, we can examine the tissues under microscope with different staining techniques. We can examine the structural change of that tissue before and after its loss of function. However, we cannot unveil some hidden functions of brain until a definite time. For instance, there would be no cellular experiments before the discovery of microscope, structure identification before the discovery of specific staining techniques.

To know the meaning of Revelation, we cannot perform experiments. The only way to understand the meaning of the writing is to ask the Author Himself.

The Parable Of The Thorns

If Jesus told us that a man was very happy after receiving his words and baptized some years later, however, he stopped to be fruitful because of the thorns around him. What do you think those thorns are referring to?

In Matthew 13: 1– 10

That same day Jesus went out of the house and sat by the lake. Such large crowds gathered around him that he got into a boat and sat in it, while all the people stood on the shore. Then he told them many things in parables, saying: "A farmer went out to sow his seed. As he was scattering the seed, some fell along the path, and the birds came and ate it up. Some fell on rocky places, where it did not have much soil. It sprang up quickly, because the soil was shallow. But when the sun came up, the plants were scorched, and they withered because they had no root. Other seeds fell among thorns, which grew up and choked the plants. Still other seeds fell on good soil, where it produced a crop—a hundred, sixty or thirty times what was sown. He who has ears, let him hear." The disciples came to him and asked, "Why do you speak to the people in parables?"

We may think that the thorns must be something bad, like our enemies, losing our job, sickness, death of a relative, imprisonment, etc. . . .

However, we are totally wrong if we think so. What is the real meaning of thorns?

In Matthew 13: 11– 23

Jesus replied, "The knowledge of the secrets of the kingdom of heaven has been given to you, but not to them. Whoever has will be given more, and he will have an abundance. Whoever does not have, even what he has will be taken from him. This is why I speak to them in parables: . . .

"Listen then to what the parable of the sower means: When anyone hears the message about the kingdom and does not understand it, the evil one comes and snatches away what was sown in his heart. This is the seed sown along the path. The one who received the seed that fell on rocky places is the man who hears the word and at once receives it with joy. But since he has no root, he lasts only a short time. When trouble or persecution comes because of the word, he quickly falls away. The one who received the seed that fell among the thorns is the man who hears the word, but the worries of this life and the deceitfulness of wealth choke it, making it unfruitful. But the one who received the seed that fell on good soil is the man who hears the word and understands it. He produces a crop, yielding a hundred, sixty or thirty times what was sown."

See. The thorns refer to **wealth** . . . and worries!

We would not have known the meaning if Jesus had not told us in Matthew 13.

Therefore the principle of explaining the Revelation in the Bible is not only a matter of knowledge but the will of the Author. Sometimes, the readers may still not understand after asking the Author. It is not that the Author does not want to tell; otherwise, He will not reveal anything in Revelation. It may just because it is not the right time for us to understand, like the understanding of cells before the discovery of the microscope or the identification of tissue structures before the intervention of specific staining techniques. As our history progresses, the meaning of Revelation may become easy to understand. It is still our responsible to keep on asking although we may not understand now.

References:

1. Barker, R.A., Barasi, S., Neal, M.J., "Association cortices: the posterior parietal and prefrontal cortex." In: *Neuroscience at a glance, international eds.* (Oxford: Blackwell Science Ltd, 1999), pp. 70-73.

Chapter 4

How Could Jesus Become Bright During the Transfiguration? (Genetics)

What Is Genetics

Genetics is the study of genes in living organisms such as bacteria, birds, fishes, humans and semi-living organisms like viruses. Before the era of genetics, we did not know why we are different from the fishes, dogs or our grandparents. Now, at least, we have some ideas that it is due to different gene components passing from our ancestors that makes us different. However, why do different genes make different morphological structures or even different IQs or EQs? There is still a very long way to go.

In 2001, the Human Genome Project (HGP)[1] published its results to that date: a 90 percent complete sequence of all three billion base pairs in the human genome (the HGP consortium published its data on the February 15, 2001, issue of the journal, *Nature*). Surprises accompanying the sequence publication were: the relatively small number of human genes, perhaps as few as 30,000; the complex architecture of human proteins compared to their similar genes with the same functions in worms and flies; and the mystery behind repeat sequences of DNA! The mapping database is available at the Genome Sequencing Center at Washington University in St. Louis [2].

We thought we knew something but in fact we do not.

From the genetic point of view, some hardly imagined miracles can have a trace.

In Matthew 17: 1–3

After six days Jesus took with him Peter, James and John the brother of James, and led them up a high mountain by themselves. There he was transfigured before them. His face shone like the sun, and his clothes became as white as the light. Just then there appeared before them Moses and Elijah, talking with Jesus.

How could Jesus' face shine? How could his clothes become as white as the light? How can I imagine this miracle?

If the above miracle is hard to imagine, may I ask: Have you seen a mouse shining green light under fluorescent light?

Scientists nowadays can use green fluorescent protein (GFP) derived from jellyfish to incorporate in newly fertilized mouse eggs genetically. The transgenic mice, once they are born, carry a protein marker in all body tissues that make them glow green under a fluorescent light. The character is a permanent feature of the animal's genome, and is carried throughout life and is inheritable by offspring [3].

All impossible things in fact are possible but it is a matter of time. Yesterday you could not imagine it but today you see it. It is unfair to say that it's impossible because you cannot imagine it. Mice can shine and Jesus, of course, can shine, too. Mice can shine because they carry the gene of green fluorescent protein (GFP) which is located normally in jellyfish. Can Jesus have some kinds of bright shining protein at the time of transfiguration due to its receiving extraordinary energy? Is it still very difficult to imagine?

The important clue whether we believe or not is not knowledge or imagination, but faith. Only after submitting ourselves can we imagine those impossible. God proves it later.

What is the difference between believing after seeing and before seeing?

In John 20: 24–29

Thomas (called Didymus), one of the twelve, was not with the disciples when Jesus came. So the other disciples told him, "We have seen the Lord!"
But he said to them, "Unless I see the nail marks in his hands and put my finger where the nails were, and put my hand into his side, I will not believe it."
Eight days later his disciples were in the house again, and Thomas was with them. Though the doors were locked, Jesus came and stood among them and said, "Peace be with you!" Then he said to Thomas, "Put your finger here; see my hands. Reach out your hand and put it into my side. Stop doubting and believe."
Thomas said to him, "My Lord and my God!"
Then Jesus told him, "Because you have seen me, you have believed; blessed are those who have not seen and yet have believed."

References:

1. The National Human Genome Research Institute: Human Genome Project (HGP) [http://www.genome.gov -assessed on 23rd Nov, 2002]

2. Genome Sequencing Centre at Washington University in St. Louis School of Medicine. [http://genome.wustl.edu/cgi-bin/ace/GSCMAPS.cgi -assessed on 23rd Nov, 2002]
3. "Caltech 336 of the California Institute of Technology." Volume II, No. 2: January 24, 2002.

Chapter 5

The Experiment by Noah (Epidemiology)

What Does The Word "Epidemiology" Mean

Epidemiology is the study of the determinants and distribution of disease frequency in human population [2]. After knowing the distribution and determinants of disease frequency, the government can reduce the disease by implementing public measures. Some scientists consider it as a branch of public health medicine. Most of the time, we do not know the agent that causes a particular disease. Does this mean that we cannot prevent that particular disease if we do not know the causing agent, for example, a virus? In the sense of epidemiology, it is not true. We can still prevent that particular disease although we have not yet known the biological or chemical agent that cause the disease.

Why is it so?

We now know that cholera, a potentially fatal diarrhoeal disease, is caused by a group of bacteria called Vibrio cholerae. It lives in contaminated water but can be easily killed by boiling for just a few seconds[1]. However, before we knew that bacteria as a cause of cholera, Snow J had prevented the disease by the method of epidemiology.

In 1853, there was an outbreak of cholera death in London. Hundreds of people were killed in several days within the United Kingdom and the most severe outbreak occurred within 250 yards of the spot where Cambridge Street joins Board Street. Snow investigated the frequency and distribution of the outbreak and found that the people using water supply from Southwark and Vauxhall Company carried a higher occurrence to those using Lambeth Company [3]. He postulated that water supplied by the Southwark and Vauxhall Company was responsible for the outbreak of cholera in London although he did not know the causing agent or the mechanism. Facing increasing pressure, that company closed and cholera decreased dramatically. Later it was found that some pipes of that company were contaminated with the cholera agent. Decades later, bacteria Vibrio cholerae was isolated and known to be the cause of cholera.

The method used by Snow was an observational method. However, in epidemiology, the gold standard method (the best method that is widely accepted) is a good clinical trial (experiment).

Who Did The First Public Health Experiment

In Genesis 8: 1–21

God remembered Noah and all the wild animals and the livestock that were with him in the ark, and he sent a wind over the earth, and the waters receded. Now the springs of the deep and the floodgates of the heavens had been closed, and the rain had stopped falling from the sky. The water receded steadily from the earth. At the end of the hundred and fifty days the water had gone down, and on the seventeenth day of the seventh month the ark came to rest on the mountains of Ararat. The waters continued to recede until the tenth month, and on the first day of the tenth month the tops of the mountains became visible.

Here Noah had done a well-planned public health experiment. It was not actually a clinical trial as it involved no human subject. However, he used very limited resources (flying birds) to test the crucial important statement or hypothesis that the land is dry.

After forty days Noah opened the window he had made in the ark and sent out a raven, and it kept flying back and forth until the water had dried up from the earth. Then he sent out a dove to see if the water had receded from the surface of the ground. But the dove could find no place to set its feet because there was water over all the surface of the earth; so it returned to Noah in the ark. He reached out his hand and took the dove and brought it back to himself in the ark. He waited seven more days and again sent out the dove from the ark. When the dove returned to him in the evening, there in its beak was a freshly plucked olive leaf! Then Noah knew that the water had receded from the earth. He waited seven more days and sent the dove out again, but this time it did not return to him.

During the days of the Great Flood, all living creatures on earth were destroyed except eight human subjects (Noah's family) and some pairs of animals. The human population was small and it was easily extinguished. After the ark rested on the mountains of Ararat, it seemed that the waters subsided. How could he test the hypothesis that the land was dried up so that he could implement a policy to go out of the ark? The resources for him to do an experiment were scarce, only walking or flying animals or his family members. He could send four family members out of the mountains to walk in four different directions and come back to him with detailed reports. He could also send dogs or other animals similarly. However, he did not. He used just a raven which could not give him a detailed report but was affordable compared to a human. The raven flew away and did not come until the water had dried up from the earth. How could he draw conclusion from this experiment? The land was dried or the raven drowned. So he sent another dove out. She came back to the ark because there was no resting place.

By the first day of the first month of Noah's six hundred and first year, the water had dried up from the earth. Noah then removed the covering from the ark and saw that the surface of the ground was dry. By the twenty-seventh day of the second month the earth was completely dry.

Now Noah knew that the dove was a reliable tool for him to carry this experiment. He waited another seven days and used this reliable tool again. The dove came back with a freshly plucked olive leaf. Noah drew the conclusion that the waters had abated from the earth (Genesis 8:11). Should he implement a policy to the population that they have to go?

No. As a policy maker to his population, he waited another seven days. He sent the dove again and this time she did not return. It was a good sign for a leader of great confidence to lead his people out as the experiment had shown that the land was dried. Although he believed that the land was already dried as he removed the covering of the ark and looked that indeed it was dry (Genesis 8:13), he did not immediately go nor made a policy to let the people go. Until he heard the Lord spoke to him, saying, "Go out of the ark, you and your wife, and your sons and your sons' wives with you. Bring out with you every living thing of all fresh that is with you: birds, and cattle and every creeping thing that creeps on the earth, so that they may abound on the earth, and be fruitful and multiply on the earth." (Genesis 8: 15–17), he implemented a policy to go.

He came out, together with his sons and his wife and his sons' wives. All the animals and all the creatures that move along the ground and all the birds — everything that moves on the earth — came out of the ark, one kind after another. Then Noah built an altar to the Lord and, taking some of all the clean animals and clean birds, he sacrificed burnt offerings on it. The Lord smelled the pleasing aroma and said in his heart: "Never again will I curse the ground because of man, even though every inclination of his heart is evil from childhood. And never again will I destroy all living creatures, as I have done."

How should a good leader implement a policy in order to do good to his people, based on his own judgment or based on scientific evidence?

In fact, in the experiment of Noah, there was still a chance that the dove did not return because of drowning or some other hazards. Even a gold standard trial can only tell us that it is of 95% confidence or 99% confidence to believe the result is true. It implies that there is always 1 or 5 % that the result is wrong from reality.

References:

1. Kumar, P., Clark, M., *Clinical Medicine.* 4th edition. (London: W. B. Saunders, 1998).
2. MacMahon, B., Pugh, T.F., *Epidemiology : Principles and Methods.* (Boston: Little, Brown, 1970).
3. Snow, J. *On the Mode of Communication of Cholera,* 2nd eds. (London: Churchill, 1855). Reproduced in Snow on Cholera. (New York: Hafner, 1965).

Chapter 6

What Is the Purpose of Sour Wine in Crucifixion? (Pharmacology)

What Is Pharmacology

Pharmacology is the study of drugs together with their mechanism, absorption, dissemination, elimination and interaction with other drugs. One of the oldest drugs that had been used for at least two thousand years is alcohol. The chemical name of ethyl alcohol is ethanol. Now we consume alcoholic beverages but no longer consider it an oral medication. However we are still using alcohol (75% ethanol) topically for skin antiseptic.

What Are The Effects Of Alcohol In Our Body

Usually half a pint of beer or a glass of wine can raise the blood alcohol concentration by 20 mg/dL[1].

- When the blood alcohol level is between 20–99 mg/dL, we may have happy sensation (euphoria) or impaired coordination.
- When the blood alcohol level is between 100–199 mg/dL, we may have poor judgment or unstable mood.

- When the blood alcohol level is between 200–299 mg/dL, we may have slurred speech or vomiting.
- When the blood alcohol level is between 300–399 mg/dL, we may have stage 1 anesthesia or memory disturbance.
- When the blood alcohol level is more than 400 mg/dL, we may have breathing failure, coma or death.

As stated above, blood alcohol level of less than 100 mg/dL may lead to euphoria. The amount required is about five glasses of wine but of course it depends very much on the health status of the subject himself. People have been using alcohol to induce this happy sensation for quite a long time, for example in wedding.

The Use Of Wine In Cana

In John 2: 1–11, Jesus Changes Water to Wine

On the third day a wedding took place at Cana in Galilee. Jesus' mother was there, and Jesus and his disciples had also been invited to the wedding. When the **wine** was gone, Jesus' mother said to him, "They have no more wine."

"Dear woman, why do you involve me?" Jesus replied, "My time has not yet come."

His mother said to the servants, "Do whatever he tells you."

Nearby stood six stone water jars, the kind used by the Jews for ceremonial washing, each holding twenty to thirty gallons.

Jesus said to the servants, "Fill the jars with water"; so they filled them to the brim.

Then he told them, "Now draw some out and take it to the master of the banquet."

They did so, and the master of the banquet tasted the water that had been turned into **wine**. He did not realize where it had come from, though the servants who had drawn the water knew. Then he called the bridegroom aside and said, "Everyone brings out the choice **wine** first and then the cheaper **wine** after the guests have had too much to drink; but you have saved the best till now."

This, the first of his miraculous signs, Jesus performed in Cana of Galilee. He thus revealed his glory, and his disciples put their faith in him.

Jesus converted water into wine, not simply wine but good wine. Water (chemical formula is H_2O) was changed to ethyl alcohol (chemical formula is CH_3CH_2OH) together with some tasty components. Wine was used to induce happy sensation in the wedding of Cana. Good wine added an extra good memory in this feast.

The Use Of Wine By Timothy

Alcohol consumption can have good or bad effect in our body. Excessive alcohol can tear the esophagus and lead to bleeding, so called the Mallory-Weiss syndrome [3]. Some diseases like pancreatitis, hepatitis and neuropathy are related to excessive drinking. However mild consumption is believed to reduce the risk of coronary heart disease nowadays. Some people, like Paul believed that mild consumption was good to the stomach. Why?

In 1 Timothy 5: 21–23

Paul told Timothy: I charge you, in the sight of God and Christ Jesus and the elect angels, to keep these instructions without partiality, and to do nothing out of favoritism. Do not be hasty in the laying on of hands, and do not share in the sins of others. Keep yourself pure. Stop drinking only water, and use a little **wine** because of your stomach and your frequent illnesses.

Paul always cared about the health of Timothy and advised him drinking not only water but some wine. Timothy must have always been busy working and having only water when he felt hungry. Although we know that stomach ulcers are caused by a type of bacteria infection called Helicobacter pylori, hunger and irregular meals contributes it too. Alcohol therefore might be good to Timothy to relieve his hunger as one gram of ethanol (ethyl alcohol) gives rise to 7 kilocalories energy and it should be more when taking other ingredients into account [2]. Wine can therefore decrease the hunger sensation of Timothy and might relieve his stomach discomfort.

Today doctors never prescribe alcohol to people who are having stomach pain as effective drugs are plentiful. The discovery of bacteria Helicobacter pylori in causing stomach and duodenal ulcers even revolutionized the concept of stress-induced ulcers. Before the era of Helicobacter, some psychologists had hundreds of stress-induced mechanisms and pathways to account for ulcer diseases. But now no one mentions them anymore.

The Use Of Wine By Jesus

Wine therefore seemed to be good for health. Did Jesus take alcohol?
Yes.

In Matthew 27: 27–34, The Soldiers Mock Jesus

What Is the Purpose of Sour Wine in Crucifixion?

Then the governor's soldiers took Jesus into the Praetorium and gathered the whole company of soldiers around him. They stripped him and put a scarlet robe on him, and then twisted together a crown of thorns and set it on his head. They put a staff in his right hand and knelt in front of him and mocked him. "Hail, king of the Jews!" they said. They spit on him, and took the staff and struck him on the head again and again. After they had mocked him, they took off the robe and put his own clothes on him. Then they led him away to crucify him.

As they were going out, they met a man from Cyrene, named Simon, and they forced him to carry the cross. They came to a place called Golgotha (which means The Place of the Skull). There they offered Jesus **wine** to drink, mixed with gall; but after tasting it, he refused to drink it.

In John 19: 28–30, The Death of Jesus

Later, knowing that all was now completed, and so that the Scripture would be fulfilled, Jesus said, "I am thirsty." A jar of **wine** vinegar was there, so they soaked a sponge in it, put the sponge on a stalk of the hyssop plant, and lifted it to Jesus' lips. When he had received the drink, Jesus said, "It is finished." With that, he bowed his head and gave up his spirit.

Why did the soldiers give Jesus wine to drink? Did they want to help Jesus as he said that he was thirty? Some people think that alcohol can be acted as antiseptic and have euphoric (happy) property and gall is bitter and therefore can distract the painful sensation of crucifixion. But alcohol can only be acted as antiseptic when used in topical mean. Why did a crucified man need alcohol to drink for antiseptic purpose? As stated above, the amount of 1–5 glasses of wine can lead to euphoria but the soldiers did not give him a full jar ["vessel" in New King James Version] of wine (John 19: 29) but soaked the sponge. Could gall really relieve or distract the pain from crucifixion?

I myself have a rather different opinion here. The sour wine with gall was not a help from the soldiers but one of the mockeries. Why?

Firstly, it was seldom mentioned in the Bible that wine should mix with sour and gall. Only wine alone had been mentioned in the wedding of Cana or in the letter where Paul had advised Timothy to take wine. From our experience, few cultures like to mix sour and gall to wine. In China, some people like to take wine from rice together with an intact gall bladder of snake. They believe that it is a good tonic and can improve health. Even so, the gall is intact otherwise it is impossible to swallow. (My parent asked me to taste once when I was young. They thought that it was good to me but I nearly vomited.) Have you eaten a fish that is so bitter because of a ruptured gall bladder during processing? Do you continue to swallow it or just regurgitate it? Of course you regurgitate it at once. It is as quick as a reflex response. Therefore I guess that it was a mock from the soldiers.

Secondly, the soldiers were all along mocking him with different methods; they stripped him and put a scarlet robe on him, twisted together a crown of thorns and set it on his head, put a staff in his right hand and knelt in front of him and mocked him, said "Hail, king of the Jews!" spat on him and took the staff and struck him on the head again and again. (Matthew 27:28–31) Why did they suddenly feel sympathy for him and give him remedy? Perhaps Luke 23:36–37 gives us some insight: They offered him wine vinegar and said, "If you are the king of the Jews, save yourself." Why did they say these words after giving him remedy?

Thirdly, why did they mix gall and sour to wine? Why not just give Jesus gall to taste? Have you smelled gall? It smells bad. But you may hardly smell the bad scent if it is in wine as its fragrance covers it. That is why cooks may use wine in cooking to hide the smell of internal organs. The soldiers wanted to hide the smell of gall so that Jesus would taste it.

Fourthly, if it was really a remedy, why did Jesus refuse it after tasting it? Because He knew that they were mocking him.

Fifthly, why was there a sour wine mixed with gall? I guess this might also be the tool for making more pain to the prisoners. Have you ever tried to stain your wound with alcohol? Yes, it causes burning pain.

I therefore believe that the sour wine mixed with gall was not a remedy for Jesus but a mock from the soldiers who spat on him.

References:

1. Clare, A.N., *Psychological Medicine.* In: Kumar, P., Clark, M., *Clinical Medicine.* 4th edition. (London: W. B. Saunders, 1998), pp. 1105–48.
2. Clark, M.L., *Nutrition.* In: Kumar, P., Clark, M., *Clinical Medicine.* 4th edition. (London: W. B. Saunders, 1998), pp. 189–216.
3. Crawford, J..M., *The Gastrointestinal Tract.* In: Cotran, R.S., Kumar, V., Collins, T. *Robins Pathologic Basis of Disease.* 6th ed. (USA: WB Saunders Co. 1999), pp.779–80.
4. Lieber, C.S., "Medical disorders of alcoholism." *New England Journal of Medicine* (1995): 333: 1058–63.

Chapter 7

The Death of Jesus (Pathology)

What Is Pathology

Pathology is the study of diseases by scientific methods, for instance, the mechanisms or process of cell illnesses and death, disease appearance and its progress in different organs or systems. Pathologists examine the gross specimen (autopsy or excised organs) together with the microscopic tissue section to diagnose a disease accurately. Tissue diagnosis is especially important in the diagnosis and treatment of cancer. Physician would like to know the type of cancer before any prescription and surgeon would like to know his excision margin is adequate enough to remove the cancer and preserve adequate functioning tissue.

The Death Process Of Jesus

Our heart has two sides: the left and right. The left pumps blood to all parts of body such as the brain, kidneys, alimentary canal, all four limbs and the heart itself except the lungs. The right side of the heart receives all blood from the above organs and pumps it to the lungs for gaseous exchange. The blood from the lungs then turns back to left side of the heart again.

Medicine In The Bible

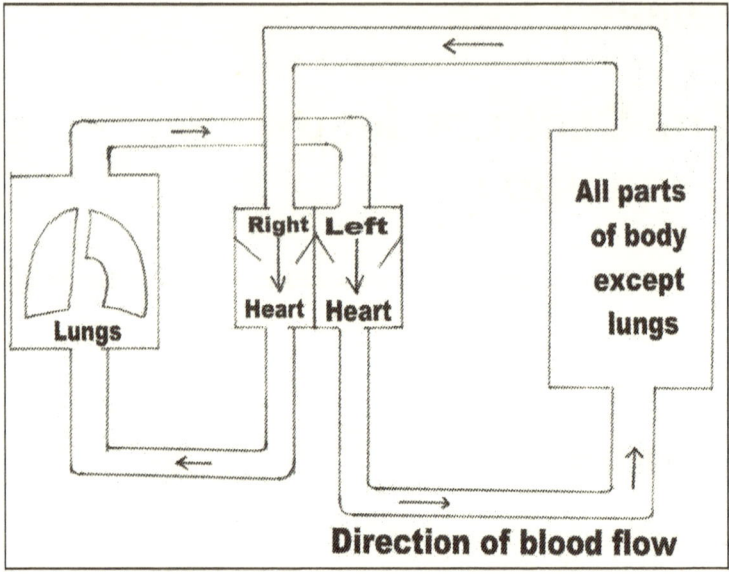

Figure 7.1 The circulation of blood

The Bible is not a book of pathology. It did not explain to us the cause of death of Jesus but the description of crucifixion was indeed clear enough for us to think about those possibilities.

In John 19: 31–34 (*The Death of Jesus*)

Now it was the day of Preparation, and the next day was to be a special Sabbath. Because the Jews did not want the bodies left on the crosses during the Sabbath, they asked Pilate to have the legs broken and the bodies taken down. The soldiers therefore came and broke the legs of the first man who had been crucified with Jesus, and then those of the other. But when they came to Jesus and found that he was already **dead**, they did not break his legs. Instead, one of the soldiers pierced Jesus' side with a spear, bringing a sudden

The Death of Jesus (Pathology)

flow of **blood and water**.

Why were there water and blood coming out from the side of Jesus? Why did Jesus die: because of blood loss or because he could not breathe? Why should the legs of a crucified man be broken in order to hasten his death? Was the blood loss quick in crucifixion?

Before answering these questions, do you know why the Jews invented the cross for death penalty? In fact, a large number of inhumane methods had been invented to torture humans since the age of our ancestors. For example, Haman made gallows seventy-five feet high for Mordecai (Esther 7:9), Nebuchadnezzar threw Shadrach, Meshach and Abednego into furnace (Daniel 3: 9–23) and Daniel into a lions' den (Daniel 6:16–17), Philistines fastened Saul's body to the wall of Beth Shan after cutting off his head (1 Samuel 31:10). The Jews in the era of Jesus might have followed these old foreign practices which had tortured them in the past and modified it to hang a living man.

The Purposes Of Crucifixion

Crucifixion has, at least, two purposes: one is to torture and the other is to insult. No hanging up in a mountain was needed if no humiliation was intended. The victim had to be hung on a piece of wood by nails, possibly three: one on each hand and the other on both feet. The reasonable position of the nail should be between the two bones of the forearm (radius and ulna bones) near the wrist because the bones of the palm are too thin to hang a heavy human and therefore easily fractured. Body positioning by palm nails might not be as "beautiful" as that by forearm nails. Moreover, a puncture of the two medium-sized arteries (radial and ulna arteries) could be easily avoided to prevent unpredictable early death. The blood loss therefore should not be quick, at least in the beginning of crucifixion. It might be evident by the two robbers on the crosses: they could still have sensible conversation while they were hanging.

In Luke 23:39–42

One of the criminals who hung there hurled insults at him: "Aren't you the Christ? Save yourself and us!"

But the other criminal rebuked him. "Don't you fear God," he said, "since you are under the same sentence? We are punished justly, for we are getting what our deeds deserve. But this man has done nothing wrong."

Then he said, "Jesus, remember me when you come into your kingdom."

What Caused The Death Of A Crucified Man

Jesus, a crucified man, died unexpectedly early on the cross. When a soldier tested whether he was truly dead by piercing his side with a spear, water and blood was coming out. Why was there water coming out?

The water should not be come from his stomach because he had not drunk the sour wine although he was thirsty. The water therefore should come from the chest. Since the heart might not contain water, the water therefore should come from the lungs. Why were the lungs congested with water?

When a man bleeds in an uncontrollable manner, his blood pressure drops and he suffers shock. The blood volume will decrease and there will be inadequate oxygen delivery to maintain the functions of the brain, heart, etc. The heart will then pump weaker and weaker and fail. The blood entering the heart from the lungs will be congested and plasma will leak out of the capillaries and small veins (venules) into the lungs. The leaking-out fluid is called transudate. It is a clear fluid-like water, containing nearly all of the blood components except red blood cells.

The "water" coming out of Jesus could therefore be the transudate of the lungs when his heart failed. The blood might have come from the heart or other great vessels inside the chest. His death probably was a result of heart failure due to uncontrolled blood loss and shock. In John 19:28, Jesus said, "I thirst" may also be a good evidence of hypovolemic shock as a patient suffering from severe fluid loss would have a thirsty sensation.

Why Did The Legs Of The Prisoners Have To Be Broken

Before we come to this question, do you know which part of the lower limb has to be broken, the thigh (femur bone) or, really, the leg (tibia or fibula bones)?

Since the muscle mass in the thigh is thick and the position is relatively high (when a man is hung and crucified), it may not be easy to break the thigh bone. The cushion effect of the thigh will make it difficult to break. The soldiers might also have difficulty in detecting whether the thigh bones were broken or not. However, the legs were different. One could easily feel the tibia (one of the leg bones) without difficulty as it is just under the skin of the shin. Very likely, the leg fracture produced would be exposed to air through the skin as the overlying skin is thin and easy to break through. This type of fracture is called open fracture. One could therefore easily determine whether the bones are broken or not.

Why should the leg bone(s) be broken in a crucified man?

In the study of trauma, three periods of peak death after injury are recognized [1].

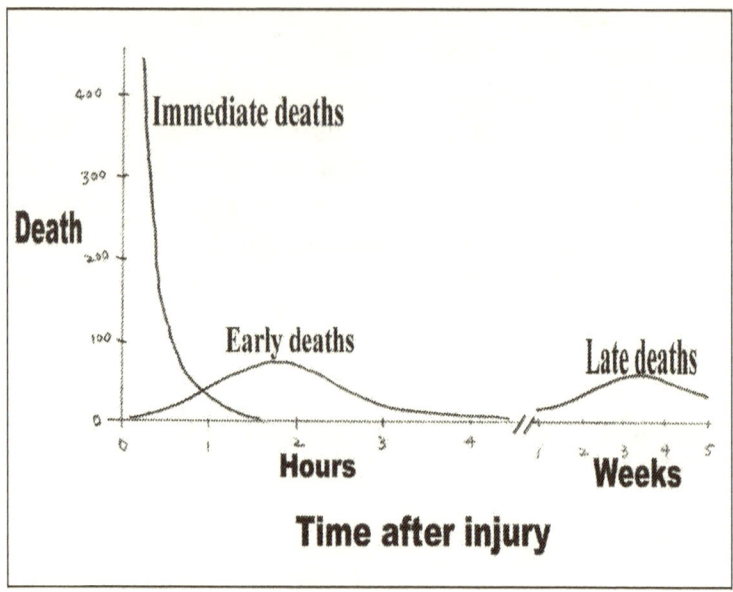

Figure 7.2 Peaks of death after injury

1. First, approximately half of all trauma-related deaths occur within **seconds or minutes** of injury and are related to lacerations of the aorta, heart, brain stem, brain, and spinal cord. Few of these patients are saved by health care systems, regardless of efficacy.
2. The second mortality peak occurs **within hours** of injury and accounts for approximately 30% of deaths, half of which are due to hemorrhage and half to central nervous system (CNS) injuries.
3. The third mortality peak includes deaths that occur from one **day** after trauma **to weeks** later. This late mortality usually is attributed to infection and multiple organ failure.

Obviously, the open fractures of the legs were not the first trauma it tended to produce which resulted in death in minutes. It was not likely to be the third trauma as the death following was too long to wait. The broken legs were likely to produce the second trauma in which death should follow in terms of hours, probably three hours.

Long bone and open fractures are well known to be fatal [3]. The induced open fracture of tibia could cause a lot of pain and further bleed in a crucified man. Because of the pain, the heart would beat even faster and the demand of oxygen would increase. Although there is an increase in the demand of oxygen and nutrients, the heart does not get adequate supply as aggravate blood loss occurs in the newly broken legs. The heart finally fails and dies [2].

Why did Jesus die so early and no leg bones were needed to be broken? Did he have extra privileges as he was the son of the God?

Obviously no, otherwise he did not need to be mocked and hung. It might have been the result of significant blood loss which happened when he was mocked. The soldiers put a thorny crown on the scalp of Jesus and whipped him. Profuse blood loss indeed could happen as the scalp is rich in blood supply.

When there were three prisoners to be crucified, the mocks should be shared either equally or go to the one who was "ugliest." Jesus was inevitably highlighted by the priests to be the "ugliest" among the three prisoners as they had hated him for so long. Therefore the mocks and whipping should be unexpectedly high and led to the "unexpected" early death by the priests. It was not a result of mercy from God as He had already turned His face away from Jesus, a sinner at that time. It was the result of extra suffering.

Jesus was alone, with beasts again from Satan and sins from us. However, he did not give up and showed to us what a perfect love is . . .

Very rarely will anyone die for a righteous man, though for a good man someone might possibly dare to die. But God demonstrates his own love for us in this: While we

were still sinners, Christ died for us. (Romans 5: 7–8)
References:

1. Hoyt, D.B., Coimbra, R., "Trauma: Introduction". In: Greenfield L.J., Mulholland, M.W., et al., *Surgery: Scientific Principles and Practice*, 3rd ed. (Philadelphia : Lippincott Williams & Wilkins, 2001).
2. Lubenow, T.R., Ivankovich, A.D., Mccarthy, R.J., "Management of acute postoperative pain". In: Barash, P.G., Cullen, B.F., Stoelting, R.K., *Clinical anesthesia*, 4th ed. (Philadelphia : Lippincott Williams & Wilkins, 1997).
3. Moehring, H.D., "Orthopedic surgery". In: Greenfield L.J., Mulholland M.W., et al. *Surgery: Scientific Principles and Practice,* 3rd ed. (Philadelphia: Lippincott Williams & Wilkins, 2001).

Chapter 8

The Ten Plagues and Microorganisms (Microbiology)

Before the era of microbiology, people believed that diseases were the result of sin. Priests therefore played a major role in healing diseases among different old cultures. After the intervention of the microscope by Van Leeuwenhoek in the seventeenth century, we see the tiny organisms that are responsible for most of the diseases.

So What Is Microbiology

Microbiology is the study of these tiny organisms, including bacteria, viruses, fungi, parasites and prions. [Note: The discovery of prions (an infectious protein without DNA) by Stanley Prusiner led him to receive the 1997 Nobel Prize in Physiology or Medicine[3].] Some people may think that microorganisms are not good creatures as they are hazardous to our health. However, among numerous types of bacteria, only a small part of them can cause diseases in human. Most of the 'good' bacteria take important part in putrefaction and recycle energy in our ecosystem. We would surely die if our Earth does not have bacteria.

The Microorganisms In Our Body

Do you know how many cells we are composed of and how many microorganisms are living in our body?

The human body normally has a large number of microorganisms which are called "normal flora." It has been estimated that the adult human is only 10% human. Why? It is because there are approximately one hundred trillion (10^{14} or 100,000,000,000,000) cells in the human adult but only ten trillion (10^{13} or 10,000,000,000,000) are human! The remaining 90,000,000,000,000 cells are the bacteria, fungi, protozoa and arthropods (small insects) that are the normal flora [1]!

In fact, most of these microorganisms are protecting us rather than harming us. They will not kill us as they need our body in order to survive. Many disease-causing bacteria can be found from food, water, insects, animals and humans. They grows in exponential curve. That means one produces two, then four, eight, sixteen, thirty-two, etc. The doubling time of E. coli (bacteria that causes diarrhea) is about twenty minutes. One E. coli can produce over 1000 progeny in three hours and over one million in seven hours [2].

The Ten Plagues In Egypt

Where can we find microorganisms in the Bible?

In fact the Ten Plagues might be a good example of microorganism outbreak. We may consider the Ten Plagues as the table shown below:

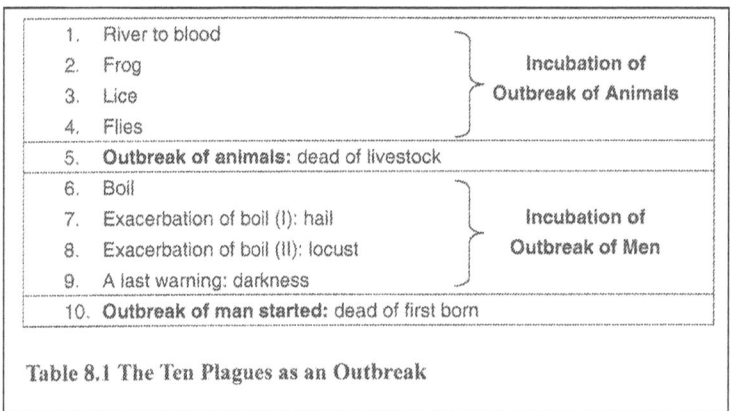

Table 8.1 The Ten Plagues as an Outbreak

The First Plague

During the first Plague, Lord said,

"By this you will know that I am the Lord : With the staff that is in my hand I will strike the water of the Nile, and it will be changed into blood. The fish in the Nile will die, and the river will stink; the Egyptians will not be able to drink its water." (Exodus 7: 17–18)

The river turned into blood and the fish died. It might have been the result of hemorrhagic disease of the fishes. The fishes leaked out blood and stained the river bloody red. In microbiology, blood is a good culture media for bacteria as it contains large amount of nutrients sustaining life. The whole Nile now became a big culture media. This unveiled the start of the later outbreak. Can you guess how many microorganisms might be produced in this big culture media of Nile?

As stated above, bacteria grow exponentially. If the growth of the bacteria in Nile is similar to that of E. coli, one bacteria will produce 5×10^{151} or

50,000,000,000,000,000,000,000,000,000,000,000,000,000,000,000,000,000,000,000,000,000,000,000,000,000,00 0,000,000,000,000,000,000,000,000,000,000,000,000,0 00,000,000,000,000,000,000,000,000,000 bacteria after seven days (Exodus 7: 25).

The Second Plague

Then the Lord said to Moses, "Go to Pharaoh and say to him, 'This is what the Lord says: Let My people go, so that they may worship Me. If you refuse to let them go, I will plague your whole country with frogs. The Nile will teem with frogs. They will come up into your palace and your bedroom and onto your bed, into the houses of your officials and on your people, and into your ovens and kneading troughs. The frogs will go up on you and your people and all your officials.' " (Exodus 8: 1–4)

The next condition to start an outbreak was: Who were responsible to bring this culture media together with the microorganisms into the land of Egypt? Great storm or flood?

No. God used the frogs. A frog is a sticky amphibian that can live in land and water. Therefore God used the frogs to carry the nutritious blood media together with those microorganisms to both man and animals on the land of Egypt. The sticky nature of the frogs now acted as a glue where the blood and germs stuck.

The Third Plague

Then the Lord said to Moses, "Tell Aaron, 'Stretch out

your staff and strike the dust of the ground, and throughout the land of Egypt the dust will become gnats.'" They did this, and when Aaron stretched out his hand with the staff and struck the dust of the ground, gnats came upon men and animals. All the dust throughout the land of Egypt became gnats. But when the magicians tried to produce gnats by their secret arts, they could not. And the gnats were on men and animals . . . (Exodus 8: 16–18)

In Egypt, most of the lands are desert and sand is therefore plentiful. The skins of man and animals might be inevitably be sticky with sand, blood and bacteria from Nile. After that, lice came. It might jump from man to man and from animal to animal. Insects are vectors of diseases and can carry microorganisms too. Those Egyptians living far away from Nile might think that the frog might not reach them effectively. Now the lice came. As these vectors jumped, bacteria and the possible diseases spread among them from coastal to inland. The spread might be slow at this phase since the lice could only jump but not fly.

The Fourth Plague

Then the Lord said to Moses, "Get up early in the morning and confront Pharaoh as he goes to the water and say to him, 'This is what the Lord says: Let my people go, so that they may worship me. If you do not let my people go, I will send swarms of flies on you and your officials, on your people and into your houses. The houses of the Egyptians will be full of flies, and even the ground where they are." . . . (Exodus 8: 20–21)

As Pharaoh hardened his heart, the rate of spread increased. Now these vectors could fly. They were flies; one of the dirtiest vectors affecting humans not only in the past but also the present.

The Fifth Plague: Outbreak Of Animals Occurred

Then the Lord said to Moses, "Go to Pharaoh and say to him, 'This is what the Lord, the God of the Hebrews, says: Let my people go, so that they may worship me. If you refuse to let them go and continue to hold them back, the hand of the Lord will bring a terrible plague on your livestock in the field — on your horses and donkeys and camels and on your cattle and sheep and goats . . . " (Exodus 9: 1–3)

As clean water source from Nile was contaminated, the Egyptians could only take water for drinking and cleaning from the uncontaminated wells. Livestock might not have been adequate cleaned as freshwater from wells was limited. They therefore developed the outbreak first. Therefore, their livestock died.

Now, Pharaoh and the Egyptians saw death, a real plague.

The Sixth Plague: Beginning Of Human Plague

Then the Lord said to Moses and Aaron, "Take handfuls of soot from a furnace and have Moses toss it into the air in the presence of Pharaoh. It will become fine dust over the whole land of Egypt, and festering boils will break out on men and animals throughout the land." (Exodus 9: 8–9)

The Ten Plagues and Microorganisms (Microbiology)

After the livestock died, the Egyptians knew that death was near for they were developing boils too. The boils might have been blisters that could burst and ulcerate. The hygiene of the whole Egypt was deteriorating. Bloodstained animals and dying animals were all around. Their wounds of boils were also all round. Human outbreak indeed could have begun at any moment. However, the heart of Pharaoh was still hard.

The Seventh Plague

Therefore, at this time tomorrow I will send the worst hailstorm that has ever fallen on Egypt, from the day it was founded till now. Give an order now to bring your livestock and everything you have in the field to a place of shelter, because the hail will fall on every man and animal that has not been brought in and is still out in the field, and they will die.... (Exodus 9: 18–19)

God sent great hailstorm to strike their boils but there was mercy. They could still hide in the house to prevent the boil from bursting. The faster the bursting of the boil, the quicker will be the spread of the infection.

The Eighth Plague

If you refuse to let them go, I will bring locusts into your country tomorrow. They will cover the face of the ground so that it cannot be seen. They will devour what little you have left after the hail, including every tree that is growing in your fields. They will fill your houses and those of all your officials and all the Egyptians—something neither your fathers nor your forefathers have ever seen from the day they settled in this land till now.... (Exodus 10: 4–6)

As the locusts came, most of the crops were eaten. The vast number of locusts could even block the sun and the land of Egypt became dark and the temperature fell. The locusts also entered the house and ruptured the boils of the Egyptians as nothing remained for them to eat. The locusts would fly and be found anywhere in the land. The Egyptians now had nowhere to hide. Their boils had to burst. Infection and an outbreak was even near. In this messy dirty land, an uncontrolled outbreak was sure to occur if there was still no respite from the locust attack.

The Ninth Plague

Then the Lord said to Moses, "Stretch out your hand toward the sky so that darkness will spread over Egypt — darkness that can be felt."... (Exodus 10: 21)

There was silence and a warning before the outbreak: the darkness. After the locusts were gone, sticky blood-stained animals were found dead or alive anywhere. Unhealed boils were still all around. Now, there was great darkness. The temperature fell.

The Tenth Plague: Outbreak Of Human Plague

So Moses said, "This is what the Lord says: 'About midnight I will go throughout Egypt. Every firstborn son in Egypt will die, from the firstborn son of Pharaoh, who sits on the throne, to the firstborn son of the slave girl, who is at her hand mill, and all the firstborn of the cattle as well. There will be loud wailing throughout Egypt — worse than there has ever been or ever will be again . . .'" (Exodus 11: 4–6)

All factors for an outbreak were now present. The whole Egypt now was dirty. Freshwater was inadequate. The weather was cold and the sky was dark. Blood and microorganisms were all around. The Egyptians had boils all over their body. An outbreak was ready. The question was: Which class of the populations would be selected as the start of the outbreak? The noble or slave? God selected the firstborn in both animals and human. The reason is unknown. It might be due to some hazardous religious rite done to the firstborn by the Egyptians.

The outbreak started quickly in the midnight.

There was no a house where there was not one dead. (Exodus 12: 30)

God punished the Egyptians and gave mercy to His people. He commanded the Israelites to eat roasted young lamb during that night. The lamb must be without blemish. They had to eat all the lamb roasted in fire but not in boiled water nor had it raw. The remains must be burnt with fire. These commands indeed were very well planned. God knew the Israelites had to travel a very long journey next morning so He commanded His people to consume young lamb without blemish. Young lamb has relatively much fat content than that of old lamb and fat yields much energy than carbohydrate (e.g., rice, potato, etc.). Therefore the Israelites could have enough energy to walk long distances. God did not want His people to get abdominal pain or diarrhea during the next morning's journey so He commanded the Israelites not to eat it raw but roasted in fire, not to boil with the contaminated water nor eat the blemish lamb. They had to burn the remaining lamb and were not allowed to bring it. Since the journey was long and they had much others to carry, for example, gold, silver and clothes, meat would also be spoiled easily in that long journey.

Pharaoh now, seeing the outbreak began, had no choice except what God had said, "**Let My people go**." If he had refused to do so, the whole Egypt would have been destroyed as the outbreak continued.

References:

1. Hart, T., Shears, P., *Diagnosis in color: Medical Microbiology.* (London: Mosby-Wolfe, 1996), pp. 1–16.
2. Levinson, W., Jawetz, E., *Examination & Board Review: Medical Microbiology & Immunology.* 5th ed. (London: Appleton & Lange 1998), pp. 13–15.
3. Press Release: The 1997 Nobel Prize in Physiology or Medicine [http://www.nobel.se/medicine/laureates/1997/press.html –assessed on 3rd September 2002]

Chapter 9

How Did Cain Kill Abel? (Forensic Medicine)

What Is Forensic Medicine

Forensic medicine is a specialized branch of study of disease and tissue injury by scientific methods which relates to the effects of trauma, poisoning, occupational hazards and natural disease within a legal framework [1]. To simplify, it is the study of the cause of death to see whether it is natural or someone has to be responsible.

When Did The First Murder Happen

In Genesis 4: 3–8 [New King James Version]

And in the process of time it came to pass that Cain brought an offering of the fruit of the ground to the Lord. Abel also brought of the firstborn of his flock and of their fat. And the Lord respected Abel and his offering, but He did not respect Cain and his offering. And Cain was very angry, and his countenance fell.

So the Lord said to Cain, "Why are you angry? And why has your countenance fallen? If you do well, will you not be accepted? And if you do not do well, sin lies at the door. And its desire is for you, but you should rule over it."

Now Cain talked with Abel his brother; and it came to pass, when they were in the field, that Cain rose up against Abel, his brother, and killed him.

Cain murdered Abel, his brother. Can we reconstruct the events surrounding the death of Abel? What caused the death of Abel? Did he die of sharp injury or blunt injury or just asphyxiation? Was there any sharp tool for killing since hard objects like copper or iron might not appear in that early human era?

From the Bible, Cain talked with Abel before killing him and when it came to pass he rose against his brother and killed him. It seemed that the event was not intentional, at least in the beginning. In this murder, the Lord did not punish Cain by death penalty but with lifelong imprisonment on an unproductive land, a cursed earth. It might be an evidence to support that it was an unintentional murder.

Metals like iron and copper were not discovered yet. Sharp tools for killing at that time were hard stones or animal bones, like Samson using a donkey's jawbone to kill the Philistines (**Judges 15:15**). If it is not likely to be an intentional murder, animal bone as a killing tool might have been less possible. Therefore Abel might have been killed by stones, fists or strangulation.

Was There Any Internal Or External Bleeding During This Murder

In Genesis 4:9, the Lord said to Cain, "What have you done? The voice of your brother's blood cries out to Me from the ground."

Therefore there should have been, at least, external

bleeding during that murder.

To reconstruct the events from the possible surrounding and what God had said, the more possible cause of Abel's death was hemorrhage after being hit by a stone, not likely to be fist or strangulation. The bleeding was so profuse that blood splattered on the ground and caused him to die.

Can the bleeding from our body be so profuse that we die? Yes, especially when the injury is on the scalp. The scalp is full of blood vessels and even blunt trauma can lead to a sharp laceration just like cutting with sharp object. The wound may be very deep and the bleeding can be very profuse.

In Acts 7: 54–60, The Stoning of Stephen

When they heard this, they were furious and gnashed their teeth at him. But Stephen, full of the Holy Spirit, looked up to heaven and saw the glory of God, and Jesus standing at the right hand of God. "Look," he said, "I see heaven open and the Son of Man standing at the right hand of God."

At this they covered their ears and, yelling at the top of their voices, they all rushed at him, dragged him out of the city and began to **stone** him. Meanwhile, the witnesses laid their clothes at the feet of a young man named Saul.

While they were **stoning** him, Stephen prayed, "Lord Jesus, receive my spirit." Then he fell on his knees and cried out, "Lord, do not hold this sin against them." When he had said this, he fell asleep.

Stephen was stoned to death and his cause of death may be similar: resulting from profuse bleeding from the scalp as the stones could cause big multiple lacerations. It might be difficult to kill a person by stoning if his head was protected.

Significant bleeding from other parts of the body could not be easily produced by stones. In the period of Jesus, Jews stoned people who had sinned especially those who committed adultery. So the whole head staining with blood was very symbolic of death and sin. That is why when they crucified Jesus, they said, "His blood be on us and on our children." (Matthew 27: 25) rather than saying "His death be on us and on our children."

By examining the wounds of Abel and Stephen, we discover murders. By examining the wounds of Jesus, we discover salvation.

References:

1. Williams, D.J., Ansford, A.J., Priday, D.S., Forrest, A.S., *Color Guide: Forensic Pathology.* 1st edition. (New York: Churchill Livingstone, 1996).

Interlude

What Is Science?

In *Longman Dictionary of Contemporary English*, Science is defined as the study of knowledge which can be made into a system and which usually depends on seeing and testing facts and stating general natural laws.

But, again what is Science and when did it begin?

In Job, chapters 38–42, Job was tested by the Lord and lost all he had. His friends talked with him and asked him why he got that experience. But in fact they did not know. Job himself had a lot of questions to ask and he surely wanted to know why. However, there was silence all along from God until it was the time.

It is very interesting to note that in the beginning, Job had a lot of questions. However, God did not give him the answers but instead even more and more questions. (Please see all these verses in the end of this chapter, it is in fact interesting.)

It seemed that God was not reasonable indeed. Why did God pose so many questions to a man who needed answers? The questions were difficult and seemed unrelated. Job of course could not answer them and indeed no one can.

Even more amazing was, after God had asked all questions, Job had the answer but no more questions. You see, the One who had answers gave questions but the one who gave questions now had answer! Their roles exchanged.

It is something like Science. When you have found something you know, you discover that more and more things you do not know simultaneously. In the end, you know that you still do not know. For example, when we found that the thing determining us is genes, we simultaneous found the questions: why are we determined by genes, how are we determined by these limited sets of genes, what other things determine us also, etc.

In Science, we have few questions in the beginning. But there are more and more difficult questions in the end, like the experience of Job.

However, Job was lucky because he ultimately got the answer. In Science, there is no absolute and ultimate answer.

When Job was in his way for finding an answer, he found more and more questions. It was in fact the beginning of Science when he humbled himself to those questions. He then opened his mind (eye) and saw God.

Science should be able to do this: humble one's mind and let him see.

Shall We Review Here What God Asked And What Job answered

The First Set Of Questions From God
(Job chapter 38–39, chapter 40: 1,2)

[1] Then the Lord answered Job out of the storm. He said:

[2] "Who is this that darkens my counsel
with words without knowledge?
[3] Brace yourself like a man;
I will question you,
and you shall answer me.

Interlude

---

⁴ "Where were you when I laid the earth's foundation?
Tell me, if you understand.
⁵ Who marked off its dimensions? Surely you know!
Who stretched a measuring line across it?
⁶ On what were its footings set,
or who laid its cornerstone—
⁷ while the morning stars sang together
and all the angels shouted for joy?

⁸ "Who shut up the sea behind doors
when it burst forth from the womb,
⁹ when I made the clouds its garment
and wrapped it in thick darkness,
¹⁰ when I fixed limits for it
and set its doors and bars in place,
¹¹ when I said, 'This far you may come and no farther;
here is where your proud waves halt'?

¹² "Have you ever given orders to the morning,
or shown the dawn its place,
¹³ that it might take the earth by the edges
and shake the wicked out of it?
¹⁴ The earth takes shape like clay under a seal;
its features stand out like those of a garment.
¹⁵ The wicked are denied their light,
and their upraised arm is broken.

¹⁶ "Have you journeyed to the springs of the sea
or walked in the recesses of the deep?
¹⁷ Have the gates of death been shown to you?
Have you seen the gates of the shadow of death?
¹⁸ Have you comprehended the vast expanses of the earth?
Tell me, if you know all this.

¹⁹ "What is the way to the abode of light?

And where does darkness reside?
20 Can you take them to their places?
Do you know the paths to their dwellings?
21 Surely you know, for you were already born!
You have lived so many years!

22 "Have you entered the storehouses of the snow
or seen the storehouses of the hail,
23 which I reserve for times of trouble,
for days of war and battle?
24 What is the way to the place where the lightning is dispersed,
or the place where the east winds are scattered over the earth?
25 Who cuts a channel for the torrents of rain,
and a path for the thunderstorm,
26 to water a land where no man lives,
a desert with no one in it,
27 to satisfy a desolate wasteland
and make it sprout with grass?
28 Does the rain have a father?
Who fathers the drops of dew?
29 From whose womb comes the ice?
Who gives birth to the frost from the heavens
30 when the waters become hard as stone,
when the surface of the deep is frozen?

31 "Can you bind the beautiful Pleiades?
Can you loose the cords of Orion?
32 Can you bring forth the constellations in their seasons
or lead out the Bear with its cubs?
33 Do you know the laws of the heavens?
Can you set up God's dominion over the earth?

34 "Can you raise your voice to the clouds

and cover yourself with a flood of water?
^{35} Do you send the lightning bolts on their way?
Do they report to you, 'Here we are'?
^{36} Who endowed the heart with wisdom
or gave understanding to the mind ?
^{37} Who has the wisdom to count the clouds?
Who can tip over the water jars of the heavens
^{38} when the dust becomes hard
and the clods of earth stick together?

^{39} "Do you hunt the prey for the lioness
and satisfy the hunger of the lions
^{40} when they crouch in their dens
or lie in wait in a thicket?
^{41} Who provides food for the raven
when its young cry out to God
and wander about for lack of food?

Job 39

^{1} "Do you know when the mountain goats give birth?
Do you watch when the doe bears her fawn?
^{2} Do you count the months till they bear?
Do you know the time they give birth?
^{3} They crouch down and bring forth their young;
their labor pains are ended.
^{4} Their young thrive and grow strong in the wilds;
they leave and do not return.

^{5} "Who let the wild donkey go free?
Who untied his ropes?
^{6} I gave him the wasteland as his home,
the salt flats as his habitat.
^{7} He laughs at the commotion in the town;

he does not hear a driver's shout.
⁸ He ranges the hills for his pasture
and searches for any green thing.

⁹ "Will the wild ox consent to serve you?
Will he stay by your manger at night?
¹⁰ Can you hold him to the furrow with a harness?
Will he till the valleys behind you?
¹¹ Will you rely on him for his great strength?
Will you leave your heavy work to him?
¹² Can you trust him to bring in your grain
and gather it to your threshing floor?

¹³ "The wings of the ostrich flap joyfully,
but they cannot compare with the pinions and feathers of the stork.
¹⁴ She lays her eggs on the ground
and lets them warm in the sand,
¹⁵ unmindful that a foot may crush them,
that some wild animal may trample them.
¹⁶ She treats her young harshly, as if they were not hers;
she cares not that her labor was in vain,
¹⁷ for God did not endow her with wisdom
or give her a share of good sense.
¹⁸ Yet when she spreads her feathers to run,
she laughs at horse and rider.

¹⁹ "Do you give the horse his strength
or clothe his neck with a flowing mane?
²⁰ Do you make him leap like a locust,
striking terror with his proud snorting?
²¹ He paws fiercely, rejoicing in his strength,
and charges into the fray.
²² He laughs at fear, afraid of nothing;
he does not shy away from the sword.

Interlude

---

²³ The quiver rattles against his side,
along with the flashing spear and lance.
²⁴ In frenzied excitement he eats up the ground;
he cannot stand still when the trumpet sounds.
²⁵ At the blast of the trumpet he snorts, 'Aha!'
He catches the scent of battle from afar,
the shout of commanders and the battle cry.

²⁶ "Does the hawk take flight by your wisdom
and spread his wings toward the south?
²⁷ Does the eagle soar at your command
and build his nest on high?
²⁸ He dwells on a cliff and stays there at night;
a rocky crag is his stronghold.
²⁹ From there he seeks out his food;
his eyes detect it from afar.
³⁰ His young ones feast on blood,
and where the slain are, there is he."

Job 40

¹ The Lord said to Job:
² "Will the one who contends with the Almighty correct him?
Let him who accuses God answer him!"

The First Answer By Job
(Job 40: 3–5)

³ Then Job answered the Lord :
⁴ "I am unworthy — how can I reply to you?
I put my hand over my mouth.
⁵ I spoke once, but I have no answer.

twice, but I will say no more."

The Second Set Of Questions From God
(Job 40: 6–24, Job 41: 1–34)

⁶ Then the Lord spoke to Job out of the storm:
⁷ "Brace yourself like a man;
I will question you,
and you shall answer me.
⁸ "Would you discredit my justice?
Would you condemn me to justify yourself?
⁹ Do you have an arm like God's,
and can your voice thunder like his?
¹⁰ Then adorn yourself with glory and splendor,
and clothe yourself in honor and majesty.
¹¹ Unleash the fury of your wrath,
look at every proud man and bring him low,
¹² look at every proud man and humble him,
crush the wicked where they stand.
¹³ Bury them all in the dust together;
shroud their faces in the grave.
¹⁴ Then I myself will admit to you
that your own right hand can save you.

¹⁵ "Look at the Behemoth,
which I made along with you
and which feeds on grass like an ox.
¹⁶ What strength he has in his loins,
what power in the muscles of his belly!
¹⁷ His tail sways like a cedar;
the sinews of his thighs are close knit.
¹⁸ His bones are tubes of bronze,
his limbs like rods of iron.
¹⁹ He ranks first among the works of God,

Interlude

---

yet his Maker can approach him with his sword.
²⁰ The hills bring him their produce,
and all the wild animals play nearby.
²¹ Under the lotus plants he lies,
hidden among the reeds in the marsh.
²² The lotuses conceal him in their shadow;
the poplars by the stream surround him.
²³ When the river rages, he is not alarmed;
he is secure, though the Jordan should surge against his mouth.
²⁴ Can anyone capture him by the eyes,
or trap him and pierce his nose?

Job 41

¹ "Can you pull in the Leviathan with a fishhook
or tie down his tongue with a rope?
² Can you put a cord through his nose
or pierce his jaw with a hook?
³ Will he keep begging you for mercy?
Will he speak to you with gentle words?
⁴ Will he make an agreement with you
for you to take him as your slave for life?
⁵ Can you make a pet of him like a bird
or put him on a leash for your girls?
⁶ Will traders barter for him?
Will they divide him up among the merchants?
⁷ Can you fill his hide with harpoons
or his head with fishing spears?
⁸ If you lay a hand on him,
you will remember the struggle and never do it again!
⁹ Any hope of subduing him is false;
the mere sight of him is overpowering.
¹⁰ No one is fierce enough to rouse him.

Who then is able to stand against me?
¹¹ Who has a claim against me that I must pay?
Everything under heaven belongs to me.
¹² "I will not fail to speak of his limbs,
his strength and his graceful form.
¹³ Who can strip off his outer coat?
Who would approach him with a bridle?
¹⁴ Who dares open the doors of his mouth,
ringed about with his fearsome teeth?
¹⁵ His back has rows of shields
tightly sealed together;
¹⁶ Each is so close to the next
that no air can pass between.
¹⁷ They are joined fast to one another;
they cling together and cannot be parted.
¹⁸ His snorting throws out flashes of light;
his eyes are like the eyelids of dawn.
¹⁹ Firebrands stream from his mouth;
sparks of fire shoot out.
²⁰ Smoke pours from his nostrils
as from a boiling pot over a fire of reeds.
²¹ His breath sets coals ablaze,
and flames dart from his mouth.
²² Strength resides in his neck;
dismay goes before him.
²³ The folds of his flesh are tightly joined;
they are firm and immovable.
²⁴ His chest is hard as rock,
hard as a lower millstone.
²⁵ When he rises up, the mighty are terrified;
they retreat before his thrashing.
²⁶ The sword that reaches him has no effect,
nor does the spear or the dart or the javelin.
²⁷ Iron he treats like straw
and bronze like rotten wood.

^{28} Arrows do not make him flee;
slingstones are like chaff to him.
^{29} A club seems to him but a piece of straw;
he laughs at the rattling of the lance.
^{30} His undersides are jagged potsherds,
leaving a trail in the mud like a threshing sledge.
^{31} He makes the depths churn like a boiling caldron
and stirs up the sea like a pot of ointment.
^{32} Behind him he leaves a glistening wake;
one would think the deep had white hair.
^{33} Nothing on earth is his equal —
a creature without fear.
^{34} He looks down on all that are haughty;
he is king over all that are proud."

The Second Answer by Job
(Job 42: 1–6)

^{1} Then Job replied to the Lord:

^{2} "I know that you can do all things;
no plan of yours can be thwarted.
^{3} You asked, 'Who is this that obscures my counsel without knowledge?'
Surely I spoke of things I did not understand,
things too wonderful for me to know.

^{4} "You said, 'Listen now, and I will speak;
I will question you,
and you shall answer me.'
^{5} My ears had heard of you
but now my eyes have seen you.
^{6} Therefore I despise myself
and repent in dust and ashes."

Chapter 10

Sleeping Disorders of Samson, David and Jesus (Medicine: Neurology)

What Comprise A Normal Sleep

Basically, there is a rapid eye movements (REM) sleep and non-REM sleep. REM sleep may be more important as it seems to restore our cognitive process. Dreaming, whether delightful or horrible, takes place during the REM sleeping [1]. Therefore, if you did not have dreams before the examination, your mind might not be clear enough.

Sleeping disturbances are in fact very common as working is not easy. Most people are suffering from excessive daytime sleepiness or poor sleep. Children are prone to sleep talk and sleep walk. Sometimes there may be night terrors and commonly nightmares, especially before the day of examination.

Excessive Sleepiness Of Jesus

Did the Bible talk about sleeping? In fact, there were many.

In Luke: 8: 22–25

One day Jesus said to his disciples, "Let's go over to the other side of the lake." So they got into a boat and set out. As they sailed, he fell **asleep**. A squall came down on the lake, so that the boat was being swamped, and they were in great danger.

The disciples went and woke him, saying, "Master, Master, we're going to drown!"

He got up and rebuked the wind and the raging waters; the storm subsided, and all was calm. "Where is your faith?" he asked his disciples.

In fear and amazement they asked one another, "Who is this? He commands even the winds and the water, and they obey him."

There is an interesting sleeping disorder called narcolepsy. People suffering from this disorder tend to have irresistible sleeping even while eating or talking! However the periods of sleep are usually short and the person can be waken up easily. They are usually suffering from sudden loss of muscle power by surprise or sleep paralysis [1].

While the disciples were sailing in the lake, Jesus fell asleep. Was he suffering from narcolepsy?

Traditionally, people thought that Jesus was pretending to sleep in order to test the faith of the disciples. It is impossible to sleep in that stormy lake. I don't know whether Jesus was really sleeping or not. However, I won't be surprised if Jesus was really sleeping at that time.

First of all, it was not likely to be narcolepsy as there was no history of sleeping while he was eating or talking as told by the Bible. He didn't seem to have sudden muscle power loss due to emotional surprise—although he is always surprised by the little faith of the disciples and ours. In fact, Jesus was really very busy at the time of his preaching. How do we know that Jesus was always busy?

In the Gospel written by his disciple, Mark, a word was repeatedly used to describe the action of Jesus, that is "again."

"A few days later, when Jesus again . . ." (Mark 2: 1)
"Once again Jesus went out . . ." (Mark 3: 13)
"Again Jesus began to teach . . ." (Mark 4: 1)

In Mark 3: 20,

Then Jesus entered a house, and again a crowd gathered, so that he and his disciples were **not even able to eat**.

It might be a good evidence to describe the busy life of Jesus during his preaching: he and his disciples were not even able to eat! Wherever Jesus was, there were people around him who wanted to be healed or who listened to his teaching. Therefore, it will not be a surprise if a man has excessive daytime sleepiness if he is as busy as that.

Before I had my driving license, I didn't believe that people can fall asleep when they drive. How could I imagine that a man can fall asleep in a dangerous speedy highway? But after I had my license, I believed that as I have slept for three times when I was driving on a speedy highway during daytime! How could it be? It was simply because of tiredness. I recognized that I was falling asleep at that time and I knew it was very dangerous. But I simply could not resist it, I was exhausted. Fortunately, there were no accidents (Now, I do not drive if I feel tired.). In fact, road traffic accidents as a result of sleep is not uncommon! The three major peaks during 24-hour period were at around 2:00 A.M., 6:00 A.M. and 4:00 P.M. Half these drivers were men under thirty years old [2].

So, Jesus might pretend to sleep in order to test his disciples but I won't be surprised if he was really sleeping at that time because of tiredness.

Sleep Disorder Of King David

Sleeping usually is productive. It may be especially true for REM sleeping as it refreshes our cognitive function. However, there are some examples of unproductive sleeping in the Bible. It occurred in David when he had been a king for some time . . .

One evening David got up from his bed and walked around on the roof of the palace. From the roof he saw a woman bathing. The woman was very beautiful, and David sent someone to find out about her. The man said, "Isn't this Bathsheba, the daughter of Eliam and the wife of Uriah the Hittite?" Then David sent messengers to get her. She came to him, and he slept with her. (She had purified herself from her uncleanness.) Then she went back home. The woman conceived and sent word to David, saying, "I am pregnant." (2 Samuel 11: 2–5)

The sleeping disorder of King David might be sleeping much more than what he really needed. Day-and-night rhythm and timekeeping is a fundamental property of all higher forms of life [3]. A normal human should not sleep much more than or much less than his biological need. However, King David seemed to sleep too much and lose his timekeeping rhythm as well as his control by the biological clock.

After King David had slept till evening, he saw from the roof something that he should not have continued to see. It was Bathsheba, the wife of Uriah, bathing. Normally, people wake up in the morning unless they need to work at night. If a man needs to work at day but still can sleep until evening, can you think of any cause? Is it his holiday? Or is he sick? We do not know whether it was the holiday of King David. But we surely know that he was not sick, otherwise he would not have slept with Bathsheba. He sinned again by killing Uriah, his loyal servant. God punished him that the sword would never depart from his house (2 Samuel 12:10). Later, King David was chased and persecuted by his son, Absalom, and there was no good sleep any more.

Sleep Disorder Of Samson

How can a sleeping man not notice that his seven braids of hair were being shaved off? It may be difficult to imagine.

Delilah asked Samson about the secret of his strength because she wanted to get money from the Philistines. He should not have told her this important and life-threatening secret but he did tell it all.

In Judges 16: 17–21

So he told her everything. "No razor has ever been used on my head," he said, "because I have been a Nazarite set apart to God since birth. If my head were shaved, my strength would leave me, and I would become as weak as any other man."

When Delilah saw that he had told her everything, she sent word to the rulers of the Philistines, "Come back once more; he has told me everything." So the rulers of the Philistines returned with the silver in their hands. Having put him to **sleep** on her lap, she called a man to shave off the seven braids of his hair, and so began to subdue him. And his strength left him.

Then she called, "Samson, the Philistines are upon you!"

He awoke from his **sleep** and thought, "I'll go out as before and shake myself free." But he did not know that the Lord had left him.

Then the Philistines seized him, gouged out his eyes and took him down to Gaza. Binding him with bronze shackles, they set him to grinding in the prison.

Samson slept on the lap of Delilah. It might have been too comfortable for him. He did not feel that his hairs were being shaved! It was not just one hair but seven braids of hair. The knife at that time might not be as sharp as that we are using now. Even if the knife was sharp, it should take some time to cut seven braids of hair. However, Samson did not notice it. He was sleeping very very deeply.

All Samson could see was black when he was sleeping on the lap of Delilah. However, when he woke up, all he could see were still black because his eyes were gouged out by the Philistines. He could never see again. However, after losing his eyes, he woke up. He 'saw' that he had sinned against the Lord. He repented and God was with him again to revenge to his enemy. The number of enemy he killed was much more than when he was alive.

References:

1. Clarke, C.R.A., *Neurological disease.* In: Kumar, P., Clark, M., *Clinical Medicine.* 4th edition. (London: W. B. Saunders, 1998).
2. Horne, J.A., Reyner, L.A., "Sleep-related vehicle accidents." *BMJ* (1995): 310: 565–567.

3. Hastings, M., "Clinical review: The brain, circadian rhythms, and clock genes." *BMJ* (1998): 317: 1704–7.

Chapter 11

Sexually Transmitted Diseases (STDs) and Repentance (Medicine)

An Example From Joseph And Mary

In Matthew 1: 24 –25

When Joseph woke up, he did what the angel of the Lord had commanded him and took Mary home as his wife. But he had no union with her until she gave birth to a son. And he gave him the name Jesus.

Here we see a man called Joseph who married his wife but had no union with her. That means Joseph did not have sex with his wife, Mary, even after they were married. How faithful was Joseph that he respected the Lord and his wife by controlling his desire for what he indeed was even justified to do. Did Joseph lack desire because he needed to flee from one place to another? Or Mary simply did not allow him to do so?

The Bible did not account for this but we know that Joseph was a normal man like us. He had at least four sons as mentioned in the Bible and they were James, Joseph, Simon and Judas (Matthew 13: 55). Although he was justified to sleep with his wife, he did not do that. He respected the Lord and his wife in such a way that he could control his desire.

Nowadays, a man sleeps with a woman even before marriage or even when he is not sure whether she will be his wife. Have we given enough respect to our spouse? Do we still fear God now?

Sexually Transmitted Diseases Today

In developed countries such as United States, the ratio of divorce to marriage is about 1:2 in 2000s [1]. Therefore in two marriages, one will end up in divorce. What do these figures mean? What is the meaning of marriage? Why do we still get married? Can we just sleep with anyone we like or just cohabit with anyone we want?

In 1981, cases of a rare cancer called Kaposi's sarcoma and an unusual chest infection called Pneumocystis carinii pneumonia were reported in the U.S. among previously "healthy" homosexual men. No one knew the reason until 1984. Scientists found out that there was an association between human immunodeficiency virus (HIV) and those strange infections. HIV was spread among homosexual men in the early 1980s but now also among heterosexuals.

According to the Joint United Nations Program on HIV/AIDS, as of the end of 2001, the following trends of the worldwide epidemic (or pandemic) of HIV are evident:

- Today, about 40 million people are living with HIV/AIDS. Of these, 37 million are adults, 19 million are women, and 3 million are children under 15.
- During 2001, AIDS caused the deaths of 3 million people, including 1 million women and 0.6 million children under 15.
- Women are becoming increasingly affected by HIV. About 50% of the 37 million adults living with HIV or

AIDS worldwide are women.
- About 95% of people with HIV now live in the developing world.

AIDS surely revolutionized the concept of sexually transmitted diseases (STDs) in our medical history. Previously STDs seldom kill, they mainly infect the genital area or sometimes other parts of our body, like late (tertiary) syphilis causing infected lesion in the nerves or big vessels which are called gummas. STDs may be curable or non-curable (viral-infected STDs) but it **rarely** kills. However, AIDS revolutionized our concept of STDs, it **always** kills. To our understanding, no one survives HIV infection up till now. The asymptomatic period after HIV infection may be 5 to 10 years before any clinical manifestation. Afterwards, the immune system breaks down and a variety of disease complex occurs. The first presentation of AIDS is also different. It appears first not on the genital area like other STDs but usually as fever, weight loss or some enlarged lymph nodes. When it does not manifest in the genital area, one can therefore hardly think of STDs.

Below is the table of some current data about STDs in the U.S. However, the figures are underestimated and the actual figures should be larger than these, as most infected people simply do not report themselves.

Sexually Transmitted Diseases	Incidence (New cases per year)	Prevalence* (People currently infected)
Chlamydia (causing urethritis)	3 million	2 million
Gonorrhea (causing urethral discharge)	0.65 million	Not Available
Syphilis (causing sex organ ulcers)	70,000	Not Available
Herpes (causing sex organ ulcers)	1 million	45 million
Human Papillomavirus (causing sex organ warts)	5.5 million	20 million
Hepatitis B (can lead to liver caner)	0.12 million	0.4 million
Trichomoniasis (causing vaginal discharge)	5 million	Not Available

* No recent surveys on national prevalence for gonorrhea, syphilis or trichomoniasis have been conducted.

Source: Cates W et al. "Estimates of the Incidence and Prevalence of Sexually Transmitted Diseases in the United States." *Sex Trans Dis* (1999) : 26 (suppl): S2-S7.

Table 11.1 Incidence and Prevalence of Sexual Transmitted Diseases in the US

What Do The Discovery Of AIDS Tell Us About

In this century, many and many people are being killed by HIV infection. Can we treat this illness or can we simply reduce the sufferings from this?

In John 8: 1–11, A Woman Caught in Adultery

Jesus went to the Mount of Olives. At dawn he appeared again in the temple courts, where all the people gathered around him, and he sat down to teach them. The teachers of the law and the Pharisees brought in a woman caught in adultery. They made her stand before the group and said to Jesus, "Teacher, this woman was caught in the act of **adultery**. In the law Moses commanded us to stone such women. Now what do you say?" They were using this question as a trap, in order to have a basis for accusing him.

But Jesus bent down and started to write on the ground with his finger. When they kept on questioning him, he straightened up and said to them, "If any one of you is without sin, let him be the first to throw a stone at her." Again he stooped down and wrote on the ground.

At this, those who heard began to go away one at a time, the older ones first, until only Jesus was left, with the woman still standing there. Jesus straightened up and asked her, "Woman, where are they? Has no one condemned you?"

"No one, sir," she said.

"Then neither do I condemn you," Jesus declared. "Go now and leave your life of sin."

Can we find cure to AIDS? It is possible but when? Even if we can find that cure, will there be new strain of lethal infection to replace AIDS? The moral standard today is surprisingly low compared to that in the Bible. Have we given enough respect to our spouse? Do we still fear God now? We all sin but not all repent. There is always chance for us to repent before Jesus. So don't be afraid. Come to Jesus.

References:

1. Kreider, R. M., Fields J. M. "Number, Timing, and Duration of Marriages and Divorces: 1996. Current Population Reports." *US Census Bureau* (2002) :70-80. [http://www.census.gov/prod/2002pubs/p70–80.pdf - assessed on 23rd Oct, 2002]
2. Centers for Disease Control and Prevention (CDC). *Semiannual HIV/AIDS Surveillance Report* (2001) [http://www.cdc.gov/hiv/stats.htm -assessed on 23rd Oct, 2002]

Chapter 12

Running and the Advice of Paul (Sports Medicine)

What Is Sports Medicine

Sports medicine encompasses many specialties such as medicine, sports and exercise. It usually deals with both the health benefits and hazards of physical activities.

We now know that regular physical activity can reduce the risk of premature mortality, coronary heart disease, hypertension, colon cancer, obesity, and diabetes mellitus. Daily, moderately intense exercise such as walking for thirty minutes yields substantial health benefits [1]. It may also protect against breast cancer, and possibly prostate, lung, and endometrial cancer [2]!

Surprisingly, physical activities are not absolutely or a hundred percent safe. Every year, 1 out of 50,000 sudden death occurred in sports. One in 20, 000 athletes have a condition that leads them to serious heart problems, and of those at risk, 10% may die suddenly or unexpectedly.

Although physical activities carry this risk, the benefits surely outweigh the hazards.

Are Our Lives Like Sports

Paul, a servant of God, has told us many times that life is just like a game, especially like running. Why?

In 1 Corinthians 9: 24–27

Do you not know that in a race all the **runners run**, but only one gets the prize? **Run** in such a way as to get the prize.
Everyone who competes in the games goes into strict training. They do it to get a crown that will not last; but we do it to get a crown that will last forever.
Therefore I do not **run** like a man running aimlessly; I do not fight like a man beating the air. No, I beat my body and make it my slave so that after I have preached to others, I myself will not be disqualified for the prize.

Why are our lives like running instead of walking?
Running is different from walking. In fact, running and boxing are both classified as high intensity activity with moderate or high dynamic demands [3]. Walking, on the other hand, is not that intensive. The risk associated is relatively small. Inevitably, life is intensive too. We see fewer and fewer smiles in our surroundings, working place and family. One has to keep in touch with his environment as everything around us is changing fast. If we do not keep on learning, it will be too late when we discover it. It seems that we have to chase the knowledge, technique and our changing world in our life.

Whether you are a Christian or not, life is really like running. It is intensive and there are risks. You have to run, but you may not win the prize.

How can we reduce the risks and intensity of running?

Paul told us, "Run in such a way as to get the prize." In fact, we will not know whether we can win until the end of the game. What we can do is run and concentrate in our lane and goal. We only know that no one can replace us and we will not regret for the rest of our life. There is no loser in the way to Heaven. Everyone will get the prize.

In Hebrews 12: 1–3

Therefore, since we are surrounded by such a great cloud of witnesses, let us throw off everything that hinders and the sin that so easily entangles, and let us **run** with perseverance the race marked out for us. Let us fix our eyes on Jesus, the author and perfecter of our faith, who for the joy set before him endured the cross, scorning its shame, and sat down at the right hand of the throne of God. Consider him who endured such opposition from sinful men, so that you will not grow weary and lose heart.

In Philippians 2:12–16

Therefore, my dear friends, as you have always obeyed — not only in my presence, but now much more in my absence — continue to work out your salvation with fear and trembling, for it is God who works in you to will and to act according to his good purpose.
Do everything without complaining or arguing, so that you may become blameless and pure, children of God without fault in a crooked and depraved generation, in which you shine like stars in the universe as you hold out the word of life — in order that I may boast on the day of Christ that I did not **run** or labor for nothing.

Running can be full of joy when we see the goal.

References:

1. Bahr, R., "Clinical review: Recent advances Sports medicine," *BMJ* (2001): 323: 328–31.
2. Centers for Disease Control and Prevention, "Surgeon general's report on physical activity and health," *JAMA* (1996): 276:522
3. Hillis, W.S., McIntyre, P.D., Maclean, J., Goodwin, J.F., McKenna, W.J., "ABC of Sports Medicine: Sudden death in sport," *BMJ* (1994): 309: 657–660

Chapter 13

Emergency of Lazarus and the Timing of Jesus (Emergency Medicine)

The Emergency Department Nowadays

What is your first impression of an emergency department? Yes. It is crowded. Overcrowding in the emergency department is an international problem and it is getting worse [1]. Some of the reasons are: lack of beds for patients admitted to hospital, lack of available specialty consultants, shortage of nursing staff, shortage of administrative and clerical support, shortage of physical space in the emergency department [2].

The Emergency Department Yesterday

In old days, maybe in the ages of Jesus, there were no emergency departments. Most of the time, patients and their relatives had to find their own cure. When people believed that disease was a result of sin, forgiveness was needed instead of cure. Priests therefore played an important role in the old 'emergency department'. They might 'cure' the rich people in their synagogues.
When patients were many but effective treatments were

scarce, people gathered quickly if there seemed to be effective treatment. That was why wherever Jesus was, there was overcrowding. It could have been much more serious than the condition of the emergency department nowadays.

In fact, the word "crowd" appears at least 125 times in the four Gospels. For examples: when Jesus saw the **crowd** around him, he gave orders to cross to the other side of the lake (Matthew 8:18); when the **crowd** saw this, they were filled with awe; and they praised God, who had given such authority to men (Matthew 9:8); such large **crowds** gathered around him that he got into a boat and sat there, while all the people stood on the shore (Matthew 13:2) ; then Jesus entered a house, and again a **crowd** gathered, so that he and his disciples were not even able to eat (Mark 3:20) ; when Jesus had again crossed over by boat to the other side of the lake, a large **crowd** gathered around him while he was by the lake (Mark 5:21) ; the next day, when they came down from the mountain, a large **crowd** met him (Luke 9:37) ; and a great **crowd** of people followed him because they saw the miraculous signs he had performed on the sick. (John 6:2)

In an overcrowded emergency department, both the doctors and patients suffer. In the overcrowded areas where Jesus was preaching, both Jesus himself and the patients suffered as there was only one doctor. Some might not be lucky enough to reach Jesus and had their diseases cured. One had to think of some methods to reach Jesus, like the lame who was carried by four men. (Mark 2:3)

Emergent Conditions Seen Nowadays And Yesterday

What are those emergency conditions seen in the emergency department nowadays? They may be acute heart diseases like coronary heart disease (CHD) and acute heart failure, drug toxicities like some anti-psychotic overdose or trauma. In Jerusalem, in those days of Jesus, traumatic and heart diseases could occur in emergency condition but drug overdose was not likely. Emergent events like toxicities might be the results of environmental hazards like heat stroke, hypothermia (low body temperature), mountain sicknesses or biological hazards like snake bite, scorpion or spider bite, eating toxic plants or mushrooms.

Most of the patients healed by Jesus seemed to be in chronic rather than acute condition for example, those lepers, paralytics, demon possessed, blind, deaf, menorrhagic, hand withered, lame, etc.

Were there any acute diseases cured by Jesus?

Yes. In Luke 4:38, Jesus rebuked the fever of Simon's mother-in-law. In Luke 22: 51, Jesus healed the high priest's servant whose right ear was cut off by his disciple. These were some examples of acute conditions healed by Jesus.

How Emergent Are Diseases Present In The Emergency Department

One of the most emergent conditions are cardiac arrests (non-beating hearts), the degree of emergency is in terms of minutes. The brain will not survive for about five minutes in complete absence of oxygen.

Life-threatening trauma or bleeding leading to shock is another real emergency. The degree is in terms of minutes to hours and largely depends on the severity of injury, the age and health status of the victims. There are also similar degrees of emergency for toxicities and they also depend on the amount taken and types of drugs.

Was The Illness Of Lazarus Emergent

In John 11: 1–44 (The Death of Lazarus)

Now a man named Lazarus was sick. He was from

Bethany, the village of Mary and her sister, Martha. This Mary, whose brother, Lazarus now lay sick, was the same one who poured perfume on the Lord and wiped his feet with her hair. So the sisters sent word to Jesus, "Lord, the one you love is sick."

When he heard this, Jesus said, "**This sickness will not end in death**. No, it is for God's glory so that God's Son may be glorified through it." Jesus loved Martha and her sister and Lazarus. Yet when he heard that Lazarus was sick, he stayed where he was for two more days.

Then he said to his disciples, "Let us go back to Judea." . . .

After he had said this, he went on to tell them, "Our friend Lazarus has fallen asleep; but I am going there to wake him up."

His disciples replied, "Lord, if he sleeps, he will get better." Jesus had been speaking of his death, but his disciples thought he meant natural sleep.

So then he told them plainly, "**Lazarus is dead**, and for your sake I am glad I was not there, so that you may believe. But let us go to him . . . "

On his arrival, Jesus found that Lazarus had already been in the tomb for four days. Bethany was less than two miles (about 3 kilometers) from Jerusalem, and many Jews had come to Martha and Mary to comfort them in the loss of their brother. When Martha heard that Jesus was coming, she went out to meet him, but Mary stayed at home.

"Lord," Martha said to Jesus, "if you had been here, my brother would not have **died**. But I know that even now God will give you whatever you ask."

Jesus said to her, "Your brother will rise again."

Martha answered, "I know he will rise again in the resurrection at the last day."

Jesus said to her, "I am the resurrection and the life. He who believes in me will live, even though he dies; and whoever lives and believes in me will never die. Do you believe this?"

"Yes, Lord," she told him, "I believe that you are the Christ, the Son of God, who was to come into the world."

And after she had said this, she went back and called her sister Mary aside. "The Teacher is here," she said, "and is asking for you." When Mary heard this, she got up quickly and went to him. Now Jesus had not yet entered the village, but was still at the place where Martha had met him. When the Jews who had been with Mary in the house, comforting her, noticed how quickly she got up and went out, they followed her, supposing she was going to the tomb to mourn there.

When Mary reached the place where Jesus was and saw him, she fell at his feet and said, "Lord, if you had been here, my brother would not have **died**."

When Jesus saw her weeping, and the Jews who had come along with her also weeping, he was deeply moved in spirit and troubled. "Where have you laid him?" he asked.

"Come and see, Lord," they replied.

Jesus wept.

Then the Jews said, "See how he loved him!"

But some of them said, "Could not he who opened the eyes of the blind man have kept this man from dying?"

Jesus, once more deeply moved, came to the tomb. It was a cave with a stone laid across the entrance. "Take away the stone," he said.

"But, Lord," said Martha, the sister of the dead man, "by this time there is a bad odor, for he has been there four days."

Then Jesus said, "Did I not tell you that if you believed, you would see the glory of God?"

So they took away the stone. Then Jesus looked up and said, "Father, I thank you that you have heard me. I knew that you always hear me, but I said this for the benefit of the people standing here, that they may believe that you sent me."

When he had said this, Jesus called in a loud voice, "Lazarus, come out!" The dead man came out, his hands and feet wrapped with strips of linen, and a cloth around his face.

Jesus said to them, "Take off the grave clothes and let him go."

When Mary and Martha told Jesus that Lazarus was sick, the degree of emergency of that illness might be in terms of days. Jesus however took no action and gave reassurance that "this illness is not unto death." Mary and Martha then went back to look after their brother and Jesus stayed two more days in the place where he was!

Then Jesus came to Judea. Lazarus had already been dead for four days. It was a misdiagnosis, misconduct in the standard of today's medical professional guidelines. Jesus must have been sued if this had happened today. Therefore Mary, although loved Jesus and had wiped his feet with her hair, might be angry with him in this event. Martha heard Jesus was coming and went to meet him but Mary was sitting in the house (John 11: 20). When Martha saw Jesus, she wept and said "Lord, if you had been here, my brother would not have died. But even now I know that . . ."

Martha told Mary secretly that "Jesus has come and is calling for you." We do not know whether Jesus had really called her as the Bible did not mention it. When Mary saw Jesus, she wept and said "Lord, if you had been here, my brother would not have died." Then the conversation stopped here and no more conversation as mentioned by the Bible. Apart from being sorrowful, Mary might be angry as well.

In fact, Mary had her right to be angry because she had completed her responsibility by telling her family doctor, Jesus, the emergent condition. However, it was totally a "misdiagnosis" leading to the death of her brother. Mary and Martha might have found another famous doctor to treat their brother if not for the false reassurance by Jesus — this sickness is not unto death . . . But all was too late. Lazarus had already been in the tomb for four days. Why? Why did Jesus not come immediately? Why did my Mary's brother need to suffer for some days?

Jesus wept and talked to Martha, "Did I not say to you that if you would believe you would see the glory of God?"

He told those people around to remove the cave stone. He called in a loud voice, "Lazarus, come out!" The dead man came out, his hands and feet wrapped with strips of linen, and a cloth around his face.

In fact, what we think as emergent may not be that "emergent" in the glory of God. He will never be late for us, just be patient.

References:

1. Derlet, R.W., Richards, J.R., "Overcrowding in the nation's emergency departments: complex causes and disturbing effects," *Ann Emerg Med* (2000): 35:63–8.
2. Fatovich, D.M., "Clinical review: Recent developments Emergency medicine." *BMJ* (2002): 324: 958–62

Chapter 14

Did Adam Have One Rib Less Than Eve? (Anesthesia)

What Is Anesthesia

Anesthesia is loss of touch and painful sensation. It facilitates operation without causing unnecessary pain and the associated muscle contraction. It is usually induced by intravenous medication and followed by gaseous drugs. Surgery without adequate anesthesia is unethical and will lead to medicolegal consequence. Unfortunately, it still occurs nowadays because of accidental equipment failure or human errors!

If Operation Without Anesthesia

Have you ever had any operation before? Did you need any local or general anesthesia for that event? If there was no anesthesia during that operation, how would it be?

I had a horrible experience from a tooth extraction when I was young. Now, I can still remember it very clearly, not because of good memory, but because it was simply very painful.

When I was ten, I had a decayed tooth that needed to be

removed. I don't know why I had that decayed tooth as I don't like candy. But it came, I had no choice. The dental surgeon injected some medication for local anesthesia (now there is topical anesthesia before that painful injection). After five minutes, he tested my sensation by pricking my gum with a needle. I said it was still painful and the medication seemed not to work. After another five minutes, he tested again but it was still painful. There were many patients outside his clinic, waiting. He said that the medication should be continued and he would like to have a try. I was a good patient and believed everything he said. Therefore, my nightmare began. I yelled and wept throughout the operation but he did not stop. I did not understand why he could do this. It took longer than usual simply because of the non-working anesthesia and my cramping mouth muscles. He sweated and so did I. Since then, I never saw him again, praise be to the Lord.

Assuredly, I tell you the truth. Operations before the nineteenth century were without anesthesia as it had not been discovered yet [3]. Patients or victims who underwent operation had to bear the pain. Some assistants around him would give "help" by pressing him firmly during the procedure. Apart from pain, surgery at that time had to overcome three basic problems: infection, bleeding and shock.

In 1846, Morton William Thomas Green used ether for dental extraction as a means of general anesthesia at Massachusetts General Hospital in the U.S. The success led to acceptance of using anesthesia in operations. Further public repute was gained when Queen Victoria used chloroform from Dr. Snow during the birth of Prince Leopold in 1857, which was eleven years later [2].

Was The First General Anesthesia Done In 1846

In Genesis 2: 18–25

The Lord God said, "It is not good for the man to be alone. I will make a helper suitable for him."

Now the Lord God had formed out of the ground all the beasts of the field and all the birds of the air. He brought them to the man to see what he would name them; and whatever the man called each living creature, that was its name. So the man gave names to all the livestock, the birds of the air and all the beasts of the field.

But for Adam no suitable helper was found. So the Lord God caused the man to fall into a **deep sleep**; and while he was sleeping, he took one of the man's ribs and closed up the place with flesh. Then the Lord God made a woman from the rib he had taken out of the man, and he brought her to the man.

The man said, "This is now bone of my bones and flesh of my flesh; she shall be called 'woman, ' for she was taken out of man." For this reason a man will leave his father and mother and be united to his wife, and they will become one flesh.

The man and his wife were both naked, and they felt no shame.

This may be the first general anesthesia. Adam was put to deep sleep when he had this first operation. He was not in coma but only in deep sleep as sleep is arousable but coma is not. If there had not been any deep sleep (general anesthesia) during this operation, Adam would have been in much pain. He might have been reluctant to have a helper, Eve. It is not even ethical to do operation without adequate anesthesia. Nowadays, the anesthetist together with the hospital will be sued if there is inadequate anesthesia during an operation.

Although it is rare nowadays, it still occurs.

Did Adam Have One Rib Less Than Eve

Some people will ask: Do men have one rib less than women since Eve was made from the rib of Adam? Most Christian medical students like to count the ribs of both men and women when they have the anatomy lesson. My colleagues and I did that before. To our surprise, it is not. All anatomy books tell us that both men and women have twelve pairs of ribs, including ten complete pairs of ribs connecting to the sternum (with or without cartilages) and two floating ribs that are only several inches long hanging on the back.

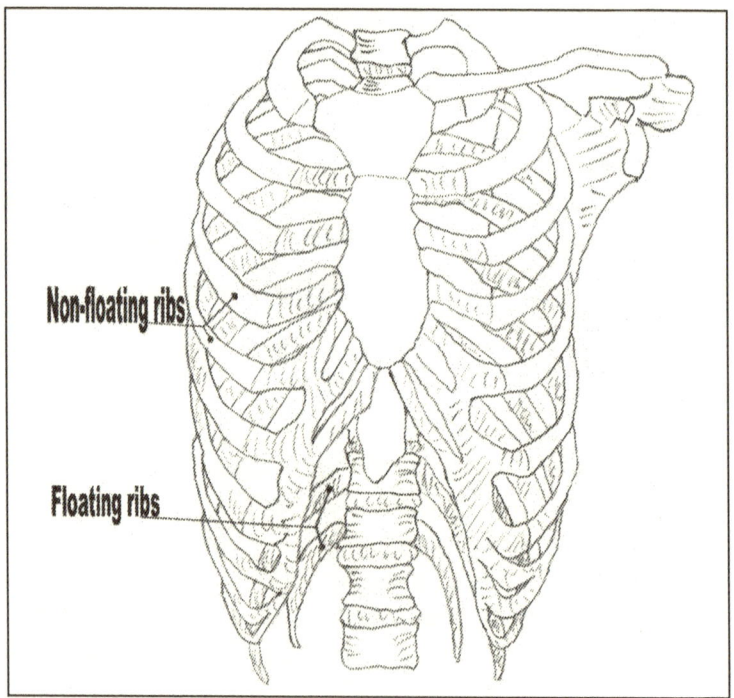

Figure 14.1 Human ribs

Did Adam Have One Rib Less Than Eve?

Some variant people have thirteen pairs of ribs because of extra cervical ribs which may sometimes cause diseases. Then why did the Bible tell us that men have one rib less? Did Adam have one rib more before the operation?

The Bible did not tell us that men have one rib less. I think originally Adam had the same twelve pairs of ribs like you and me and Eve. But before they sinned or before they ate the fruits from the Tree of Knowledge of Good and Evil, the body of Adam was perfect, not been cursed yet. The immune system of Adam was also perfect and so was the regeneration power inside him. There was no death in his body. The cells therefore will not die although there may be injury. There was no programmed cell death (apoptosis). The rib removed from Adam simply regrew and it made his body restore its state before the operation. There may not even be a scar if the generation power was perfect.

However, it was not the same after they sinned. There is programmed cell death (apoptosis). The immune system changed and death followed. The Bible used the word: separation. Degeneration and death begins. It affects all parts of our body, our brain, vessels, joints, heart, ovary, etc. Some studies found that about 1% of people by age sixty-five will get dementia and the prevalence will increase up to about 70% when one attains his age of ninety-five or older [4]. Degeneration is not only a recognized condition in the elderly but also in the youth. Nowadays, scientists have found that fatty streak, believed to be the precursors of atherosclerosis, appear in the vessels of some children even less than one year and all children older than ten years [1]!

In fact, all of us are programmed to die. Only through Jesus can we survive and live again.

References:

1. Schoen, F.J., Cotran, R.S., *Blood Vessels*. In: Cotran, R.S., Kumar, V., Collins, T., *Robbins Pathologic Basis of Disease*, 6th eds. (Philadelphia: WB Saunders Co, 1999), pp. 493–542.
2. Langford, R.M., Budd, K., "Anaesthesia and pain relief." In: Russell R.C.G., Williams, N.S., Bulstrode, C.J.K., *Bailey & Love's : Short Practice of Surgery.* 23rd ed. (New York: Oxford University Press Inc. 2000), pp. 74–87.
3. Margotta R., *Anaesthesia.* In: *The Hamlyn History of Medicine,* 1st ed. (London: Reed International Books Ltd, 1996), pp. 144–149.
4. Fratiglioni, L., De Ronchi, D., Aguero-Torres, H., "Worldwide prevalence and incidence of dementia". *Drugs Aging.* (1999): Nov.15(5):365–75.

Chapter 15

Circumcision and the Intelligence of God (Surgery)

The Most Commonly Performed Operation

Do you know what is the most commonly performed operation nowadays? Undoubtedly, circumcision is one of the most commonly done operations nowadays. It is not only one of the most commonly performed surgeries but also the earliest operation done by human as documented in Bible. (The first operation was performed by God: He opened the chest of Adam and took out a rib to make Eve.)

All Descendants Of Abraham Needed To Circumcise

Why did all descendants of Abraham need to circumcise?

In Genesis 17 : 1–14 (The Covenant of Circumcision)

When Abram was ninety-nine years old, the Lord appeared to him and said, "I am El-Shaddai (meaning God Almighty); walk before me and be blameless. I will confirm my covenant between me and you and will greatly increase your numbers."
Abram fell face down, and God said to him, "As for

me, this is my covenant with you: You will be the **father of many nations**. No longer will you be called Abram (meaning exalted father); your name will be Abraham (meaning father of many), for I have made you a father of many nations. I will make you very fruitful; I will make nations of you, and kings will come from you. I will establish my covenant as an everlasting covenant between me and you and your descendants after you for the generations to come, to be your God and the God of your descendants after you. The whole land of Canaan, where you are now an alien, I will give as an everlasting possession to you and your descendants after you; and I will be their God."

Then God said to Abraham, "As for you, you must keep my covenant, you and your descendants after you for the generations to come. This is my covenant with you and your descendants after you, the covenant you are to keep: Every male among you shall be **circumcised**. You are to undergo **circumcision**, and it will be the sign of the covenant between me and you. For the generations to come every male among you who is eight days old must be **circumcised**, including those born in your household or bought with money from a foreigner — those who are not your offspring. Whether born in your household or bought with your money, they must be **circumcised**. My covenant in your flesh is to be an everlasting covenant. Any uncircumcised male, who has not been **circumcised** in the flesh, will be cut off from his people; he has broken my covenant."

Why did God command Abraham to be circumcised as a confirmation of His covenant? What are the benefits of circumcision to all descendants of Abraham?

It is, in fact, a very interesting and clever command from

God. As we know, one of the promises to Abraham was to make his descendants as many as possible and be a great nation. Abraham however had no offspring at that time. Can circumcision increase the number of offspring so as to increase the chance of being a great nation?

The Benefits Of Circumcision

Today, many evidences have shown that circumcision can decrease the change of male penile wart (a sexually transmitted disease) and the associated penile cancer [1]. The reduced rate of penile wart is especially true in male with multiple sexual partners which was a very common practice in the time of Abraham. (Sarah even commended Abraham to sleep with her maidservant, Hagar.) Some studies even found that circumcision can protect male from HIV infection, penile carcinoma, urinary tract infections, and ulcerative sexually transmitted diseases [4]. It can also reduce the rate of female cervical cancer [2]! Nowadays, cervical cancer is one of the leading causes of deaths in women in their reproductive age. Cervical smear to detect and treat this cancer earlier is important in modern public health measure. The occurrence of abnormality as detected by cervical smear can be as high as 3–11% [3].

As stated above, circumcision actually decreases many sex organ diseases both in men and women, especially in the old days where there was no condom for the prevention of sexually transmitted diseases and multiple sexual partners was common.

How important is it to decrease the illnesses of the sex organ or even the associated death rate in a population? Was it related to the covenant of God? Was it easy for Abraham to become a great nation at that moment? What could Abraham do to increase his number of offspring? Remember that he had only one son, Isaac when he died.

Circumcise To Increase The Number Of Offspring

It is the intelligence of God because the number of offspring produced will be more in those circumcised compared to those uncircumcised. In a population where having multiple sexual partners is accepted, circumcision improved the genital health status of both men and women. The healthier the populations' reproductive status, the more frequent intercourse occurs. More offspring will be produced to compensate the early death in old days. Through this method, descendants from Abraham outnumbered other population and had a higher chance to form a nation.

In Exodus 1: 6–10

Now Joseph and all his brothers and all that generation died, but the Israelites were fruitful and multiplied greatly and became exceedingly **numerous**, so that the land was filled with them.
Then a new king, who did not know about Joseph, came to power in Egypt. "Look," he said to his people, "the Israelites have become much too **numerous** for us. Come, we must deal shrewdly with them or they will become even more **numerous** and, if war breaks out, will join our enemies, fight against us and leave the country."

The above scripture may be another evidence to show that the number of offspring produced by the Israelites was faster than those by the Egyptians. Were the sons of Abraham healthier compared with the Egyptians? Was the death rate lower among the descendants of Abraham but higher among the Egyptians?
No.

Numerous studies tell us that the health status is proportional to wealth. Poor people have more diseases while rich people have less. So, how can the Israelites be numerous when they were slaves in the land of Egypt?

It is surely the intelligence of Almighty God and the covenant with Abraham.

References:

1. Schoen, E.J., Oehrli, M., Colby, C.J., Machin, G. "The Highly Protective Effect of Newborn Circumcision Against Invasive Penile Cancer." *Pediatrics 2000*; 105 (3): e36. [Electronic article]
2. Castellsague, X., Bosch, F.X., Munoz, N., Meijer, C.J.L.M., Shah, K.V., de Sanjose, S., Eluf-Neto J., Ngelangel C.A., Chichareon, S., Smith, J.S., Herrero, R., Moreno, V., Franceschi, S., for the International Agency for Research on Cancer Multi-center Cervical Cancer Study Group. "Male Circumcision, Penile Human Papillomavirus Infection, and Cervical Cancer in Female Partners." *New Eng J Med* 2002 ; 346 (15): 1105–1112.
3. Centers for Disease Control and Prevention (CDC). Results from the National Breast and Cervical Cancer Early Detection Program, October 31, 1991–September 30, 1993. *Morbidity & Mortality Weekly Report (MMWR)* 1994; 43(29): 530–534
4. Moses, S., Bailey, R.C. , Ronald, A.R. "Male circumcision: assessment of health benefits and risks." *Sexually Transmitted Infections* 1998; 74(5): 368–373

Chapter 16

The Demon-Possessed Man in Gerasenes (Surgery: Transplantation)

Transplantation In The Bible

While Jesus was still speaking, a crowd came up, and the man who was called Judas, one of the Twelve, was leading them. He approached Jesus to kiss him, but Jesus asked him, "Judas, are you betraying the Son of Man with a kiss?" When Jesus' followers saw what was going to happen, they said, "Lord, should we strike with our swords?" (Luke 22: 47–49)

Then Simon Peter, who had a sword, drew it and struck the high priest's servant, **cutting off his right ear**. (The servant's name was Malchus.) Jesus commanded Peter, "Put your sword away! Shall I not drink the cup the Father has given me? (John 18: 10–11) No more of this!" And Jesus **touched** the man's ear **and healed him**. (Luke 22: 51)

What Is Transplantation

The 1990 Nobel Prize in Physiology or Medicine was given to Joseph E. Murray for the discoveries that have enabled the development of organ and cell transplantation into a method for the treatment of human disease [7].

Murray discovered how rejection following organ transplantation in man could be handled. He successfully transplanted a kidney between identical twins for the first time. He showed that patients with terminal kidney disease could be cured by transplantation of kidneys obtained from dead persons. The field was also open for transplantation of other organs such as liver, pancreas and heart.

Transplantation using an organ from the same species is called allograft, different species: xenograft, same person: autograft. For example, using pig heart valve to replace damaged human heart valve is an example of xenograft transplantation. Recently, some scientists are even talking about whole organ transplants from genetically modified pigs [1]. Donating part of our liver to save others is an example of allograft transplantation. Jesus curing the right ear of Malchus is the earliest example of autograft transplantation. However, it seemed that the patient did not give thanks to his doctor after this successful operation.

The Organs Can Be Transplanted Now

Up to now, most of the organs can be used to transplant. For instance, liver, kidney, heart, lung, pancreas, cornea, bone marrow transplantation, etc. Nearly all parts below the head are the targets for recent or future transplants. How about the brain? Can our brain be transplanted too? If the answer is yes, what will be the identity of a young man receiving a brain from an old lady? A young man or an old lady?

Fortunately, this complex issue has not occurred yet. Brain transplantation seems to be remote from the time being. Although some animal studies have tried to demonstrate some inspiration, most of them have not been successful [2, 4]. The neural tissues died after three months of transplantation [4]. Some doctors have tried to put adrenal tissues rather than brain tissues into the brain in treating Parkinson's disease but the transplanted adrenal tissue was found dead later [3]. Recently, scientists and doctors are talking about the possibility of using fetal brain tissue (from a dead baby) in treating degenerative brain diseases such as Parkinson's disease [5, 6]. The result is still controversial.

Can Brain Be Transplanted

Years ago, a TV program showed an interview with a neurosurgeon who had successfully transplanted a whole brain from monkey A to monkey B. Unfortunately, I could not find the source now. The video of monkey B who underwent the transplantation was shown but the monkey died later after the operation. It was also clearly shown that the monkey seemed to be a bit confused about its surroundings. It lay in bed with a head splint and bandages but its eyes could move around and blink.

We may ask: Can this experiment be reproduced by other neurosurgeons again? Or can this experiment be reproduced in other animals or even humans? To answer the question: "What will a young man's personality be after being transplanted with an old lady's brain?" we may find some clues from below:

In Mark 5: 1–10, (The Healing of a Demon-Possessed Man)

They went across the lake to the region of the Gerasenes. When Jesus got out of the boat, a man with an evil spirit came from the tombs to meet him. This man lived in the tombs, and no one could bind him any more, not even with a chain. For he had often been chained hand and foot, but he tore the chains apart and broke the irons on his feet. No one was strong enough to subdue him. Night and day among the tombs and in the hills, he would cry out and cut himself with stones.

When he saw Jesus from a distance, he ran and fell on his knees in front of him. He shouted at the top of his voice, "What do you want with me, Jesus, Son of the Most High God? Swear to God that you won't torture me!" For Jesus had said to him, "Come out of this man, you evil spirit!"

Then Jesus asked him, "What is your name?"

"My name is Legion," he replied.

When the man with the evil spirit of Gerasenes was asked about his name, he did not reply with his own name but with "Legion," the name of the evil spirit. Therefore the identity of the body does not belong to the fresh but the spirit. One may reasonably think that if a young man is transplanted with the brain of an old lady, he will not be the young man anymore although his appearance is the same. He will become the old lady, with his previous body.

The above statement will only be right if our spirit is situated in the brain. But if not, what will happen? Will that transplantation end up with a living flesh without spirit, like the transplanted monkey B although it could still blink and move its eyes?

If our spirit is really situated in the brain, which part or parts of the brain can we find our spirit? If the spirit is situated in tissue A of the brain, what will it be when we transplant only half of tissue A? How about one-third or one-fourth of it? How about leaving some tissue A of the recipient and put in some tissue A from the donor? Shall we produce half the spirit or a mixed-spirit person? If mixed, who will dominate? The one with more tissue or the one with more will power?

Transplantation indeed is an important breakthrough in the medical history. Patients' lives can be prolonged by a donated organ. However, the donated organ may be rejected afterward or get failure after some years. There is no permanent replacement of an organ so that we can live forever. Only through the way of Jesus can our whole body be 'transplanted' to an immortal figure.

References:

1. Weiss, RA. "Clinical review: Science, medicine and the future Xenotransplantation." BMJ 1998; 317: 931–4.
2. Lehman, MN, Silver, R, Gladstone, WR, Kahn, RM, Gibson, M, Bittman EL. "Circadian rhythmicity restored by neural transplant. Immunocytochemical characterization of the graft and its integration with the host brain." *J Neurosci.* 1987 Jun.7(6):1626–38.
3. Peterson, DI, Price, ML, Small, CS. "Autopsy findings in a patient who had an adrenal-to-brain transplant for Parkinson's disease." *Neurology.* 1989 Feb.39(2 Pt 1):235–8.
4. Ignacio, V, Collins, VP, Suard, IM, Jacque, CM. "Survival of astroglial cell lineage from adult brain transplant." *Dev Neurosci.* 1989;11(3):175–8.
5. Le Belle, JE, Svendsen, CN. "Stem cells for neurodegenerative disorders: where can we go from here?" *BioDrugs.* 2002;16(6):389–401.
6. Redmond, DE Jr. "Cellular replacement therapy for Parkinson's disease—where we are today?" *Neuroscientist.* 2002 Oct;8(5):457–88.
7. Press Release: The 1990 Nobel Prize in Physiology or Medicine [www.nobel.se/medicine/laureates/1990/press.html –assessed on 14th Oct 2002]

Chapter 17

No Let-up in Heavy Menstrual Bleeding (Gynecology)

A Bleeding Women

In Capernaum, when Jesus was on his way to heal the little daughter of Jairus, a ruler of synagogue, he met a poor bleeding woman. The dying little girl was twelve years old while the bleeding woman had been bleeding for twelve years. Therefore, the sick woman had bled since the birth of that little daughter. She had suffered a lot under the care of many doctors and had spent all she had, yet instead of getting better she grew worse. Moreover, she was considered unclean by the law. (Leviticus 15: 25–27)

In Mark 5: 27–29,

When she heard about Jesus, she came up behind him in the crowd and touched his cloak, because she thought, "If I just touch his clothes, I will be healed." Immediately her bleeding stopped and she felt in her body that she was freed from her suffering.

So, what was the cause of her bleeding illness? Was that blood really menses or just coming from another site?
It seemed that the Bible did not mention about the

nature of the bleeding. However, one of the most common and well-known causes of prolonged bleeding in women is profuse menstrual bleeding. It does occur nowadays. The reason of her menstrual bleeding was unknown but it was not likely to be cancer of the reproductive organ otherwise she could not have survived for twelve years.

Theoretically, no one would know she was bleeding and unclean if she did not tell anybody. The profuse blood loss only occurs during menstrual periods, no matter if it was regular or very irregular. The only abnormalities between the periods of heavy menstrual flows might be those illnesses resulting from low hemoglobin level such as paleness, easy tiredness, shortness of breath and small physique. In the Western world today, profuse menstrual bleeding is the most common cause of iron-deficiency anemia [1]. The symptoms can be any combination as mentioned above.

When the heavy menstrual bleeding came, it was difficult to hide it and she found it embarrassing. There was no tampon in the past and we do not know what the substitute was when there were menstrual periods. The sudden occurrence of profuse menstrual blood loss stained the clothes and caused odorous smell. The odorous smell was a result of bacterial overgrowth as blood itself is a very nutritious food. She might also faint if the blood loss was really heavy. However, if she hid herself with many clothes, no one could notice her blood stained clothes or even smelled it. The woman therefore might be accustomed to hiding herself in the crowd for she did not like people to stigmatize her as unclean.

However, Jesus pointed her out of the crowd.

In Mark 5: 30–34

At once Jesus realized that power had gone out from him. He turned around in the crowd and asked,

No Let-up in Heavy Menstrual Bleeding (Gynecology)

"**Who** touched my clothes?"

"You see the people crowding against you," his disciples answered, "and yet you can ask, 'Who touched me?'"

But Jesus kept looking around to see who had done it. Then the woman, knowing what had happened to her, came and fell at his feet and, trembling with fear, told him the whole truth. He said to her, "Daughter, your faith has healed you. Go in peace and be freed from your suffering."

Now, she was pointed out of the crowd by Jesus and she had to come out by herself. Jesus did not like her to hide herself anymore. Why should a woman doing something right still have to hide?

"No one lights a lamp and **hides** it in a jar or puts it under a bed. Instead, he puts it on a stand, so that those who come in can see the light. For there is nothing **hidden** that will not be disclosed, and nothing concealed that will not be known or brought out into the open." (Luke 8: 16–17)

It is also important to note that although she had been sick for twelve years, had spent all she had, people around her did not like her because she was unclean, and she was weak and pale, she had not given up. She still had faith in Jesus. She might not have reached Jesus easily if he had walked quickly. However, she made it. She touched the clothes of Jesus and got healed immediately. She did not need to spend even a dollar.

So, **don't give up,** my friend. Just ask the Lord for help. He is surely listening.

Do you remember the praying method told by Jesus?

Then Jesus told his disciples a parable to show them that they should **always pray and not give up**. He said: "In a certain town, there was a judge who neither feared God nor cared about men. And there was a widow in that town who kept coming to him with the plea, 'Grant me justice against my adversary.'

"For some time he refused. But finally he said to himself, 'Even though I don't fear God or care about men, yet because this widow keeps bothering me, I will see that she gets justice, so that she won't eventually wear me out with her coming!'"

And the Lord said, "Listen to what the unjust judge says. And will not God bring about justice for his chosen ones, who cry out to him day and night? Will he keep putting them off? I tell you, he will see that they get justice, and quickly. However, when the Son of Man comes, will he find faith on the earth?" (Luke 18: 2–8)

References:

1. Prentice, A. "Clinical review: Fortnightly Review, medical management of Menorrhagia." *BMJ* 1999; 319: 1343–5

Chapter 18

The Pregnancies of Sarah and Rebekah (Obstetrics)

What Is Pregnancy

Pregnancy is a female condition of having a developing fetus in the body. A pregnant woman may have the following symptoms or complaints [4]:

1. Cessation of menstruation
2. Vomiting or nausea
3. Breast enlargement with tenderness
4. Darkening of the areola
5. Frequency of urination
6. Tiredness

Women have menstrual cycles in her reproductive age, and therefore it is easy for them to suspect pregnancy when there is a missed period. If a woman has already passed her reproductive years, how can she notice the symptoms and signs of pregnancy? As we know, menopause is a normal phenomenon. Women approaching fifty (maybe earlier) will face their climacteric period and their menstrual cycles will stop gradually or abruptly. Finally, there will be no more menstrual flow.

How Could Sarah Know That She Was Pregnant

After God re-promised that Sarah would have a son, she laughed because she thought that it was some kind a joke: "Shall I surely bear a child, since I am old?' (Genesis 18: 13). She might think: "Can an old woman have her period again and give birth?"

Sarah, whom God promised would have a child, had already passed her menstrual years (Genesis 18: 12). So, how could Sara know that she was pregnant? She had no menses at all when God reassured her a son. How could she experience a "missed period" for her to suspect a pregnancy?

Sarah might experience some of the symptoms of pregnancy listed above but would she suspect that they were the result of conception? Would Sara have nausea and vomiting? Perhaps, but this non-specific symptoms might not lead her to think of the possibility of pregnancy. Nausea and vomiting might be just the result of food poisoning or bowel disorder. Would Sara have breast enlargement or darkening of the areola again? Perhaps, but for a post-menopausal old lady like her, these changes might not be very marked and lead her to think of pregnancy. Would Sara have frequency of urination because of the enlarging womb? Perhaps, but for every old lady, frequency of urination is common. Sometimes they may even have incontinence.

Therefore how did Sarah know that she was pregnant?

She might notice that her abdomen was bulging gradually. However, she might not think that it was the result of pregnancy as progressive bulging of abdomen could be due to other diseases such as tumor of bowel or ovary. The feelings of Sarah might not be easy as she did not know whether it was the promise of God coming true or she simply had a disease. The feelings might persist until the first movements inside her abdomen. It usually involves about eighteen to twenty weeks of gestation for women in their first conception [1]. When she noticed the movement of the baby, she could be sure that it was not a disease but a promise coming true. All the worries were replaced by laughs, the name of her son. (Isaac means "he laughs")

Sarah really laughed this time, not because of the "joke" of God but His promise.

Sarah said, "God has brought me **laughter**, and everyone who hears about this will **laugh** with me." And she added, "Who would have said to Abraham that Sarah would nurse children? Yet I have borne him a son in his old age." (Genesis 21: 6–7)

The Pregnancy Problems Of Rebekah

It seemed that most women in the house of Abraham had some kinds of pregnancy problems. Sarah conceived when she was old while Rebekah seemed to suffer a lot because of twin pregnancy.

In Genesis 25: 21–26,

Isaac prayed to the Lord on behalf of his wife, because she was barren. The Lord answered his prayer, and his wife, Rebekah, became pregnant. The babies jostled each other within her, and she said, "Why is this happening to me?" So she went to inquire of the Lord.

The Lord said to her, "Two nations are in your womb, and two peoples from within you will be separated; one people will be stronger than the other, and the older will serve the younger."

When the time came for her to give birth, there were **twin** boys in her womb. The first to come out was red, and his whole body was like a hairy garment, so they named him Esau. After this, his brother came out, with his hand grasping Esau's heel, so he was named Jacob. Isaac was sixty years old when Rebekah gave birth to them.

How Did Rebekah Suffer Because Of Twin Pregnancy

Rebekah was a brave girl; she followed the servant of Abraham to an unknown place to marry a person she had not seen. However, she still asked the Lord for help because of the pregnancy, the sufferings might be very severe. Compared to singleton pregnancy, women of twins (like Rebekah) will have increased nausea and vomiting, increased weight gain and the associated back pain and leg swelling, increased anemia and the associated symptoms of tiredness and breathless, increased urinary tract infection with painful urination, increased frequencies of fetal kicking and pregnancy-induced hypertension [2, 3].

In fact, twin pregnancy is not easy for humans. It was no wonder why Rebekah felt difficult as she had to bear the twins for several months.

References:

1. Bovone, S, Pernoll, ML. "Normal Pregnancy & Prenatal Care." In: DeCherney, AH., Nathan, L. *Current Obstetric & Gynecologic Diagnosis & Treatment*. (USA: McGraw-Hill Inc., 2003).
2. Bush, M., Pernoll, M.L., "Multiple Pregnancy." In: DeCherney, AH., Nathan, L. *Current Obstetric & Gynecologic Diagnosis & Treatment*. (USA: McGraw-

Hill Inc., 2003).
3. Spellacy, W.N., "Multiple Pregnancy." In: Scott, JR, Di Saia, PJ, Hammond, CB, Spellacy, WN. *Danforth's Obstetrics and Gynecology*, 8th ed. (Philadelphia: Lippincott Williams & Wilkins, 1999).
4. Stabile, I., Chard, T., Grudzinskas, G., *Clinical Obstetrics and Gynecology*. 2nd edition. (London: Springer, 2000).

Chapter 19

Bones and Pop Music (Orthopedics)

What Is Orthopedics

Orthopedics is the study of the prevention and correction of diseases of the bones, joints, tendons, ligaments, muscles and its associated soft tissues. The management of orthopedic illnesses can be accomplished by medical or surgical means. For example, osteoarthritis can be managed by different pain killer medications or operation by replacing an artificial joint. With the help of those metallic and silicon joints, patients regain their mobility for some years.

The Association Of Bone And Pop Music

Have you listened to pop music? Do you know what the most commonly found organs in those songs or lyrics are?

Yes, they are the heart, lips, mind or soul. For example, she breaks my heart, he breaks her heart, I kissed your lips, she kissed his lips, he kissed her lips, etc. However, it is something different in the old songs of Hebrew. Do you know what is the organ commonly found in Psalms (a collection of old Hebrew song) but not in today's lyrics?

Yes. It is bone. For example: Be merciful to me, Lord, for I am faint; O Lord, heal me, for my **bones** are in agony.

(Psalm 6:2); I am poured out like water, and all my **bones** are out of joint. My heart has turned to wax; it has melted away within me. (Psalm 22:14); I can count all my **bones**; people stare and gloat over me. (Psalm 22:17); My life is consumed by anguish and my years by groaning; my strength fails because of my guilt and my **bones** grow weak. (Psalm 31:10); When I kept silent, my **bones** wasted away through my groaning all day long. (Psalm 32:3); Because of your wrath there is no health in my body; my **bones** have no soundness because of my sin. (Psalm 38:3); My **bones** suffer mortal agony as my foes taunt me, saying to me all day long, "Where is your God?" (Psalm 42:10); Let me hear joy and gladness; let the **bones** you have crushed rejoice. (Psalm 51:8)For my days vanish like smoke; my **bones** burn like glowing embers. (Psalm 102:3); Because of my loud groaning I am reduced to skin and **bones**. (Psalm 102:5); They will say, "As one plows and breaks up the earth, so our **bones** have been scattered at the mouth of the grave." (Psalm 141:7)

Bones In Lyrics

Why did David and other composers of Psalms like to use the word "bone" in their lyrics?

Songs help us to share and release our feelings and emotions. Most of the times, people like to use different words to express the feelings of pain, sorrow and sadness. A bone, in fact, is a very suitable organ to express the feeling of pain. It is not a non-living structure, as many people think, it is a living organ that has both building up and breaking down processes. There are numerous nerve endings in the cover layer of bones called periosteum.

Do you know what the most common cause of disabilities among adult in the U.S. is?

It is arthritis.

Heart and lungs diseases only comprise about 8% and 5% of disability. Arthritis however, contributes nearly 18% of disability in adult. It is almost three times that for heart and lungs diseases [1].

Arthritis is a leading cause of disability in most developed countries. It is comprised of different diseases and conditions. One of the most common causes of arthritis is osteoarthritis (a wear-and-tear degenerative joint disease, especially in the elderly). The common symptoms include pain, stiffness, and swelling in or around the joints. About 43 million Americans or one of every six people have arthritis. As people get older, the number will increase dramatically. By 2020, almost one in five will be affected by arthritis and their daily activities will be limited [2].

The Lyrics Today

It is therefore not surprising to find that the word "bones" frequently appeared in the songs of Psalms. Israel, in the days of King David, might have been more "developed" than those countries around her and the life span of the Israelites might have increased as well. As people lived longer, arthritis became a major disability among the population, like all developed countries such as the U.S. and European Union today.

It may be rather surprising to notice that the words used in the lyrics today are not comprehensive as compared to those in the past.

References:

1. Centers for Disease Control and Prevention (CDC). "Prevalence of disabilities and associated health conditions among adults." (United States:1999.) *MMWR Morbidity & Mortality Weekly Report* 2001; 50: 120.

2. Centers for Disease Control and Prevention (CDC). "At a Glance. Targeting Arthritis: Public Health Takes Action," 2002.

Chapter 20

How Could Nicodemus Be Born Again? (Pediatrics)

What Is Pediatrics

Pediatrics is the study of children's health. Who are the children then? Pediatricians usually take care of the children from birth (sometimes fetus as consulted by obstetricians) to age eighteen. However, the upper limit of age varies from place to place and it may be the result of hospital policy, academic interest or other reasons. Therefore it is not surprising to see a man at his thirties still followed up in the pediatric department.

What Are The Characteristics Of Children In Jesus' saying

In Matthew 18:3

And he said: "I tell you the truth, unless you change and become like little **children**, you will never enter the kingdom of heaven.

In Mark 10:14

> When Jesus saw this, he was indignant. He said to them, "Let the little **children** come to me, and do not hinder them, for the kingdom of God belongs to such as these."

Obviously, Jesus did not define "children" by chronological age otherwise no adult can enter the kingdom of God. The definition of children in the kingdom of God therefore may have different criteria. What are they?

In John 3: 1–15 (Jesus Teaches Nicodemus)

> Now there was a man of the Pharisees named Nicodemus, a member of the Jewish ruling council. He came to Jesus at night and said, "Rabbi, we know you are a teacher who has come from God. For no one could perform the miraculous signs you are doing if God were not with him."
> In reply Jesus declared, "I tell you the truth, no one can see the kingdom of God unless he is born again."
> "How can a man be born when he is old?" Nicodemus asked. "Surely he cannot enter a second time into his mother's womb to be born!"
> Jesus answered, "I tell you the truth, no one can enter the kingdom of God unless he is born of water and the Spirit. Flesh gives birth to flesh, but the Spirit gives birth to spirit. You should not be surprised at my saying, 'You must be born again.' The wind blows wherever it pleases. You hear its sound, but you cannot tell where it comes from or where it is going. So it is with everyone born of the Spirit."
> "How can this be?" Nicodemus asked.
> "You are Israel's teacher," said Jesus, "and do you

not understand these things? I tell you the truth, we speak of what we know, and we testify to what we have seen, but still you people do not accept our testimony. I have spoken to you of earthly things and you do not believe; how then will you believe if I speak of heavenly things? No one has ever gone into heaven except the one who came from heaven — the Son of Man. Just as Moses lifted up the snake in the desert, so the Son of Man must be lifted up, that everyone who believes in him may have eternal life."

Can we enter our mother's womb again so as to be reborn? If yes, how? What, in fact, does a baby do inside his mother's womb?

In fact, a baby does a lot of things inside his mother's womb. He develops his own organs and learns how to use them.

■ At his 23rd–24th day, he develops his heart and begins to beat, irregular at first but very regular later [1].
■ At his 25th–27th day, his optic vesicle (a part of the eye) appears. Of course he cannot see because his brain is not well developed yet and there is not much to see inside the dark water of the womb [1].
■ At his 28th–30th day, his arm bud (primitive arm) appears. There is no movement at first, only later. A woman in her first pregnancy usually perceives the first fetal movement at 18–20 weeks of pregnancy [1].
■ At his 31st–34th day, his leg bud (primitive leg) appears. There is also no movement at first, only later [1].
■ By the 5th week, his three main subdivisions of brain: forebrain, midbrain, and hindbrain are evident [1].
■ By the 16th week of gestation, his diaphragm is formed [1].
■ His external sex organs begin to develop at 4 weeks after conception [4].

For a fetus to be ready to be born, it already has all necessary organs although they may not be fully functional. For example, he already has at least thirty breathing movements in every thirty minutes despite the absence of air inside his lungs [3]. The movements are only the preparation exercises to his lifelong breathing after birth.

His heart is beating but not like the heart of adult. It only functions as a single pump. It will soon act as two pumps in series after birth, like the heart of adult, one pumps to the lungs while the other pumps to the rest of body.

He already has eyes but does not see as his eye nerves and brain have not yet fully developed. There is not much to see in the dark environment inside his mother's womb, too.

He has ears but does not hear accurately as his middle ears are filled with fluid and so is his environment, inside the womb.

He has limbs but there are little movements as there is little space inside the womb.

He has vocal cords and a tongue but does not speak as there is no air in his lungs.

How Can I Be Born Again? I Am Old

Nicodemus asked Jesus, "How can I be born again to eternal life? I am old."

The fetus in his mother's womb may ask his mother, "How can I be born and survive in human environment? I am different from other human adult. I will surly die." His mother may tell him then, "You must be born in order to survive and you will surely die if you are not born. There will not be enough food for you in this womb and I will die, too. So you must be born in order to live."

Jesus may tell us the same thing about this world, "The world we are living will come to an end and die. We must be born again in order to survive in eternity."

"But how?" we may ask.

Jesus told Nicodemus that only through water and spirit will one be born again. Water may imply repentance and spirit trust in Jesus. Nicodemus, however, puzzled, "How can it be?" Jesus replied to him, "One may not understand now but one must have the ability to experience it." He used the wind as an example.

The mother may tell her fetus how he can breathe by his lungs and speak by his mouth, how he can see by his eyes and hear by his ears. She may also explain to her son the function of the womb and why it will fail in providing enough food for him later. But her son may surely find it difficult to understand. The son may ask, "How can it be? How can I see with my eyes, hear with my ears, breathe with my lungs?" The mother may tell her son, "You do not need to understand it all otherwise it will be too late for you. You will surely experience it after you are born. Don't be afraid. Just believe. I am your mother."

How can Nicodemus understand all the experience of rebirth and how can we understand it?

References:

1. Bernfield, M.R., "Developmental Biology." In: McMillan, JA, DeAngelis, CD, Feigin, RD, Warshaw, JB. *Oski's Pediatrics: Principles and Practice*. (USA: Lippincott Williams & Wilkins, 1999).
2. Behrman, R.E., Kliegman, R.M., Jenson, H.B., *Nelson Textbook of Pediatrics*, 16th eds. (Philadelphia: W.B. Saunders Co., 2000).
3. Stabile, I., Chard, T., Grudzinskas, G., *Clinical Obstetrics and Gynecology*. 2nd edition. (London: Springer, 2000).
4. Craven, C., Ward, K., "Embryo, fetus, and placenta:

normal and abnormal." In: Scott, JR, Di Saia, PJ, Hammond, CB, Spellacy, WN. *Danforth's obstetrics and gynecology*, 8th ed. 1999. (Philadelphia: Lippincott Williams & Wilkins, 1999).

Chapter 21

The Healing of Blindness (Ophthalmology)

What Is Ophthalmology

Ophthalmology is the study of eyes, the visual pathway and its diseases. Apart from biological system of an eye, knowledge of optics and electromagnetic wave is also important in the understanding of how we see. For simplicity, we see because we have eyes and a brain. A newborn baby in fact sees thing vaguely. He perceives the world mainly through vague images and sound of his caretaker and the surrounding environment. Through the eyes, we see in fact two images but our brain puts it in one and generates stereotypic 3-D images [5].

Why Does Someone See A Girl As Beautiful But Others Do Not

In 1 Samuel 16: 1, 5–7 (Samuel Anoints David)

The Lord said to Samuel, "How long will you mourn for Saul, since I have rejected him as king over Israel? Fill your horn with oil and be on your way; I am sending you to Jesse of Bethlehem. I have chosen one of his sons to be king." . . .

Then he consecrated Jesse and his sons and invited them to the sacrifice. When they arrived, Samuel saw Eliab and thought, "Surely the Lord's anointed stands here before the Lord."

But the Lord said to Samuel, "Do not consider his **appearance** or his **height**, for I have rejected him. The Lord does not look at the things man looks at. Man looks at the **outward appearance**, but the Lord looks at the heart."

God told us that we see people as handsome or beautiful by two criteria. First is the appearance (attractive big eyes or sleepy small eyes; straight nose or saddle nose) and the second is the physical build (tall or short; robust or fragile; muscular or elegant). Samuel, although a prophet, a judge and a priest of the Lord, still saw people through his eyes and brain. However, God told him that He looks at the **heart** of people, not his outward appearance. It is because as time passes by, all outward appearance of man gets worse but only the heart can get better if God is with him.

How can we train ourselves to look at people's hearts but not their outward appearance?

Recently, Harvard Medical School and Massachusetts Institute of Technology (MIT) developed an artificial retinal transplant. This new and expensive device is invented to help some people suffering from non-congenital blindness. A tiny chip responding to light signals is implanted to the retina. The chip may bypass the diseased retina and transmits light signals through the healthy eye nerves to the brain [1-4]. Some blind people will now be able to see.

The Healing of Blindness (Ophthalmology)

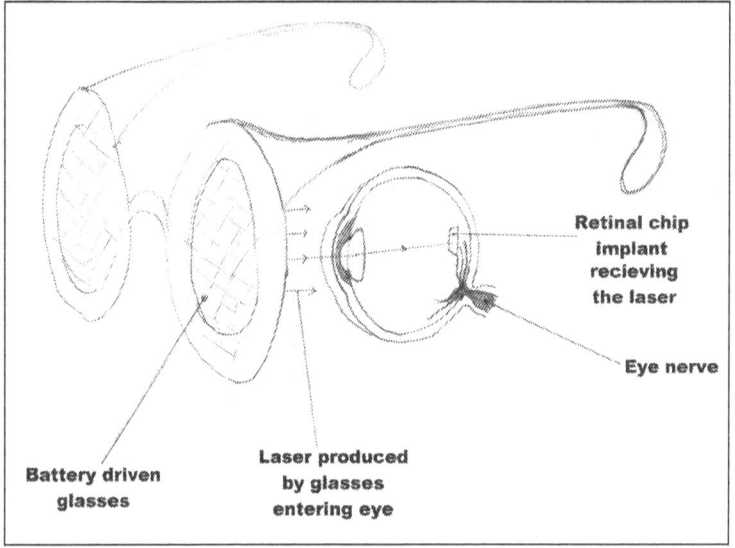

Figure 21.1 **Retinal implant of the eye**

However, can a man born blind see again? In the medical point of view, it is impossible unless the baby is immediately treated after he was born, the sooner the better. Why? It is because the eyes of a baby are not yet fully developed when he is born [6]. The later development of his eyes may take months or years and it requires the continuous stimulation of different meaningful light patterns. The stimulation of different meaningful light patterns during his growth must also be incorporated with their unique meanings that can be interpreted by his brain. For instance, the light stimulus of a candy must be associated with a sweet experience in order to create meaningful pictures created by his eyes and brain. A man born blind can hardly tell us the shape of a star no matter how hard you try to explain it. When a child is born blind, his retina will lack light stimulus to grow. It will hardly grow again once this growing phase pass.

A Man Born Blind

However, if a man born blind can really see again, what will he think? How will he interpret the outside world? What will be the first thing he would want to see?

In John 9: 1-34, (Jesus Heals a Man Born Blind)

As Jesus went along, he saw a man **blind** from birth. His disciples asked him, "Rabbi, who sinned, this man or his parents, that he was born **blind**?"

"Neither this man nor his parents sinned," said Jesus, "but this happened so that the work of God might be displayed in his life. As long as it is day, we must do the work of him who sent me. Night is coming, when no one can work. While I am in the world, I am the light of the world."

Having said this, he spit on the ground, made some mud with the saliva, and put it on the man's eyes. "Go," he told him, "wash in the Pool of Siloam" (this word means Sent). So the man went and washed, and came home seeing.

His neighbors and those who had formerly seen him begging asked, "Isn't this the same man who used to sit and beg?" Some claimed that he was.

Others said, "No, he only looks like him."

But he himself insisted, "I am the man."

"How then were your eyes opened?" they demanded.

He replied, "The man they call Jesus made some mud and put it on my eyes. He told me to go to Siloam and wash. So I went and washed, and then I could see."

"Where is this man?" they asked him.

"I don't know," he said.

The Healing of Blindness (Ophthalmology)

They brought to the Pharisees the man who had been **blind**. Now the day on which Jesus had made the mud and opened the man's eyes was a Sabbath. Therefore the Pharisees also asked him how he had received his sight. "He put mud on my eyes," the man replied, "and I washed, and now I see."

Some of the Pharisees said, "This man is not from God, for he does not keep the Sabbath."

But others asked, "How can a sinner do such miraculous signs?" So they were divided.

Finally they turned again to the **blind** man, "What have you to say about him? It was your eyes he opened."

The man replied, "He is a prophet."

The Jews still did not believe that he had been blind and had received his sight until they sent for the man's parents. "Is this your son?" they asked. "Is this the one you say was born **blind**? How is it that now he can see?"

"We know he is our son," the parents answered, "and we know he was born **blind**. But how he can see now, or who opened his eyes, we don't know. Ask him. He is of age; he will speak for himself." His parents said this because they were afraid of the Jews, for already the Jews had decided that anyone who acknowledged that Jesus was the Christ would be put out of the synagogue. That was why his parents said, "He is of age; ask him."

A second time they summoned the man who had been **blind**. "Give glory to God," they said. "We know this man is a sinner."

He replied, "Whether he is a sinner or not, I don't know. One thing I do know. **I was blind but now I see!**"

Then they asked him, "What did he do to you? How

did he open your eyes?"

He answered, "I have told you already and you did not listen. Why do you want to hear it again? Do you want to become his disciples, too?"

Then they hurled insults at him and said, "You are this fellow's disciple! We are disciples of Moses! We know that God spoke to Moses, but as for this fellow, we don't even know where he comes from."

The man answered, "Now that is remarkable! You don't know where he comes from, yet he opened my eyes. We know that God does not listen to sinners. He listens to the godly man who does his will. Nobody has ever heard of opening the eyes of a man born blind. If this man were not from God, he could do nothing."

To this they replied, "You were steeped in sin at birth; how dare you lecture us!" And they threw him out.

Sometimes, Jesus healed the blind by just a word and did not need them to do anything. For example, he healed blind Bartimaeus in Jericho (Mark 10: 46-52) and two blind men in Capernaum (Matthew 9: 27–31). He just touched them and made them see without any washing.

Why did some blind persons need to do something before they were cured but some did not? What made their methods of cure different?

Do you think that a doctor will treat patients with common cold with the same medication? Of course, no. It is simply because different people need different treatments. An old fragile man with common cold may need antibiotic while a young athlete with the same common cold may not need it.

The Healing of Blindness (Ophthalmology)

Why Did The Man Born Blind Need To Wash His Eyes Before He Could See

If Jesus had healed him right there, what would he have seen afterwards? It might be the compassionate face of Jesus, his surrounding people (all were strangers), the sky and the land. What more? How about his own face?

Some years ago, I had seen on TV a young girl with both her eyes operated in a developing country because of some kinds of cataract. After the nurse undressed her eye bandages, she was delighted when she saw her family. Her parent "introduced" each family member to her and finally they gave her a mirror to see herself. The girl took the mirror at once to see her face for a long time. She explored her face with the mirror carefully. She looked at her face at different views before the mirror. The operation was successful.

For the man who was born blind as mentioned above, his parents left him already. He lived alone, begging for money. As he did not have any family member, who would be the first one he would want to see after he gained his vision? The one who healed him? Perhaps true. But Jesus may think that knowing himself is more important than seeing his appearance. Therefore, like the parent of the little girl on TV, Jesus might want him to see his own face first. It might be difficult to find a mirror in the past, especially for the poor. Water, however, was much easier. Jesus sent him to the Pool of Siloam. Jesus might not want the blind man to lose his faith on his way to wash it. He made some mud and spat it to his eyes. It was indeed dirty and sticky. The blind man had to wash it anyway because of the stickiness and dirtiness. After he washed his eyes, the first one he saw was **himself**. He might see other people and their reflection through the water afterwards.

Who Was The Next One The Blind Man Wanted To See? His Parents?

No, his parent had left him all along like a stranger, even after he gained his sight! His parent could recognized him but he could not know who his parent were if they kept silent in front of him. It was because the blind man has never seen his parent before. Therefore, he wanted to see Jesus, the one who healed him.

Later, when the man saw Jesus again, he **saw** the appearance of Jesus — **using his eyes**.

Jesus asked him, "Do you believe in the Son of God?" The man answered, "Who is He? Lord, that I may believe in Him." Jesus said to him, "You have both **seen** Him and it is He who is talking to you." Then the man said, "Lord, I believe." And he worshiped Him. (John 9: 35–38)

After knowing who Jesus was, not just the one who healed him, he **saw** the Son of God — **using his heart**.

The blind now sees. Can we?

References:

1. Wyatt, J.L., Rizzo J.F., "Ocular Implants for the Blind." *IEEE Spectrum*. 1996; 33: 47–53.
2. Rizzo, J.F., Wyatt, J.L., "Prospects for a Visual Prosthesis." *Neuroscientist*. 1997; 3: 251–262.
3. Rizzo, J.F., Wyatt, J.L., "Retinal Prosthesis." In: Berger, JW, Fine, SL, Maguire, MG. *Age-Related Macular Degeneration*, eds. (Mosby, St. Louis, 1998), pp. 413–432.
4. Rizzo, J.F., Loewenstein, J., Wyatt, J.L., "Development

of an Epiretinal Electronic Visual Prosthesis: The Harvard-Medical Massachusetts Institute of Technology Research Program." In: *Retinal Degenerative Diseases and Experimental Theory*, (Kluwer Academic/ Plenum Publishers, 1999), pp. 463–470.
5. Kansk, J.J., "Strabismus." In: *Clinical Ophthalmology*, 3rd ed. (Oxford: Butterworth-Heinemann, 1997), pp. 427–454.
6. Westheimer, G., "Visual Acuity." In: Moses, R.A., Hart, W.M. *Adler's Physiology of the eye: clinical application.* 8th ed. (USA: Mosby, 1987), pp. 415–428.

Chapter 22

Hear the End of Age (ENT)

What Is Otorhinolaryngology

Otorhinolaryngology is a medical term. It means the study of ear, nose and throat (ENT), including the vocal cord and part of the airway. The medical term indeed is not difficult for "oto" means ear, "rhino" means nose and "laryngo" means larynx. Externally, it seems that ears and nose are separated. But in fact, they are not. A canal called Eustachian's tube connects the middle ear and the nose inside. That is why when someone has common cold and blockage of that tube, he may get ear symptoms or hearing impairment. Chewing gum or swallowing can relieve the pressure symptom of the ear when a plane is taking off.

The First Meaning Of Hearing

Sound, in fact, is a longitudinal wave of frequencies between 20 Hz to 20000 Hz. Most of the sounds are in the frequencies between 2000 to 6000 Hz like electric drills, pop stars singing, motor racing, etc. If an animal (let's say, a giraffe) produces sound out of this range, we cannot hear it although we have ears. We may think that this animal is mute but, in fact, they are not. Sound wave moves our eardrum and the inner ear fluids together with the hair cells inside. The hair cells transmit electrical impulses to our brain and then we hear. There are different kinds of hair cells for different pitches of sound: thinner hair cells for high-pitched sounds while thick hair cells for low-pitched sounds.

Degenerative deafness is common nowadays. It affects approximately 23% of the population between 65 and 75 years of age and 40% of the population older than seventy-five years of age [2]. People suffering from this illness may find it difficult to communicate with others. It may be simply because other people do not want to communicate with them. Their social life and even normal daily living may be severely affected. They may develop depression as they find themselves isolated.

Have you met old people, perhaps not as old as we think, who have degenerative hearing difficulties? Their family members may suspect that they are not really deaf because sometimes they hear but sometimes they do not. Why is this so?

For an old man whose deafness is due to advancing age, the hearing deficit, in fact, does not equally affect all low and high-pitched sound. The one that is mainly affected is the high-pitched sound because the damaged part is mainly the thinner hair cells in the beginning. Do you know why the first damage part is the thin hair cells? Have you played a guitar? How many strings are there? Which string is frequently broken and why?

The reason behind may be the same with a guitar with a broken string. There are six strings in a classic guitar. The most frequently broken string is the thinnest string (the lowest string when you are holding a guitar). The thin hair cells detecting high-pitched sounds are easily damaged when one becomes old. An old man therefore will be more deaf in high-pitched sounds but less deaf in medium and low-pitched sounds in the beginning. Next time when you talk to an old man or lady with degenerative deafness, you can just communicate with them by speaking a bit louder and not to let your voice reach a high pitch. It is not that difficult to communicate with them once you know the trick.

Can A Deaf Man Hear Nowadays

In modern medicine, the typical answer is always "Yes, but only for some people" Today's medicine is indeed advanced in some aspects. Some deaf can regain their hearing by an artificial implant: the cochlear implant. The artificial hearing aid is implanted in a deaf patient who still has a functioning auditory nerve. (Artificial nerve is developing to bypass the diseased auditory nerve now.) It will replace the diseased cochlea and transmit sound impulses to the brain. The quality of sounds, however, is not that clear. The patient therefore still needs to be intelligent enough and able to read lips during conversation [1].

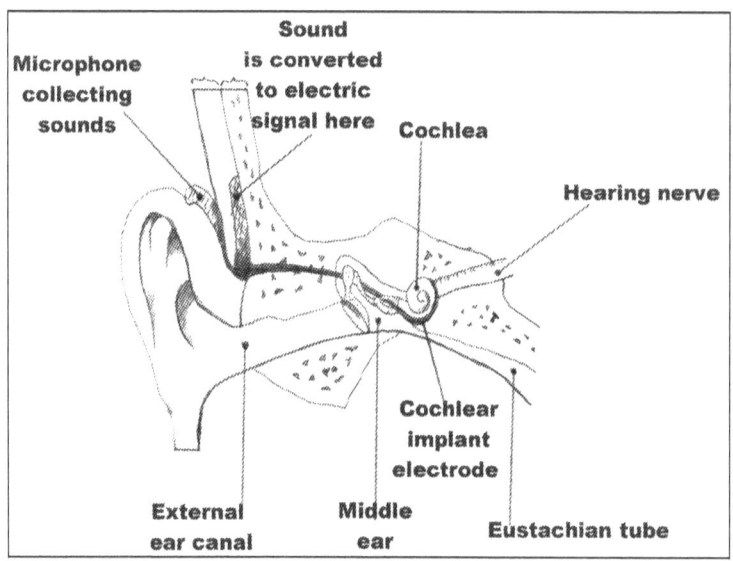

Figure 22.1 The cochlear implant for hearing loss

In Mark 7: 31–37 (*The Healing of a Deaf and Mute Man*)

Then Jesus left the vicinity of Tyre and went through Sidon, down to the Sea of Galilee and into the region of the Decapolis. There some people brought to him a man who was deaf and could hardly talk, and they begged him to place his hand on the man.

After he took him aside, away from the crowd, Jesus put his fingers into the man's ears. Then he spat and touched the man's tongue. He looked up to heaven and with a deep sigh said to him, "Ephphatha!" (which means, "Be opened!"). At this, the man's ears were opened, his tongue was loosened and he began to speak plainly.

Jesus commanded them not to tell anyone. But the more he did so, the more they kept talking about it. People were overwhelmed with amazement. "He has done everything well," they said. "He even makes the deaf **hear** and the mute speak."

Jesus healed the deaf-mute man and made him hear and speak. What were the first words he spoke? Why was there no description of those words that were first spoken by him?

It was because Jesus had already taken him aside to treat. Why? There was no answer. It might be that the surrounding was so crowded and noisy. Jesus wanted the first sound he heard was his own voice saying, "Can you hear me? Show me your tongue now." This sound would surely be the most unforgettable sound for the rest of his life. The first words he spoke might be, "I . . . I . . . I can." But was it true? Only God knows.

The Second Meaning Of Hearing

Hearing can have a second meaning. It has not only the biological component but also has the meaning of understanding that should be proven by the following action. Jesus told us not to be a foolish man as the flood is near. Faith without deeds is dead. (James 2:20)

But everyone who **hears** these words of mine and does not put them into practice is like a foolish man who built his house on sand. (Matthew 7: 26).

This is why I speak to them in parables: "Though seeing, they do not see; though **hearing**, they do not hear or understand. In them is fulfilled the prophecy of Isaiah: 'You will be ever **hearing** but never understanding; you will be ever seeing but never perceiving.'" (Matthew 13: 13–14).

Hearing is therefore the first step of taking appropriate action.

The Third Meaning Of Hearing

Hearing can have a third meaning. It reveals the communication nowadays. Why?

In Matthew 24:1–8 (Signs of the End of the Age)

Jesus left the temple and was walking away when his disciples came up to him to call his attention to its buildings. "Do you see all these things?" he asked. "I tell you the truth, not one stone here will be left on another; every one will be thrown down."

As Jesus was sitting on the Mount of Olives, the disciples came to him privately. "Tell us," they said, "when will this happen, and what will be the sign of your coming and of the end of the age?"

Jesus answered: "Watch out that no one deceives you. For many will come in my name, claiming, 'I am the Christ,' and will deceive many. You will **hear** of wars and rumors of wars, but see to it that you are not alarmed. Such things must happen, but the end is still to come. Nation will rise against nation, and kingdom against kingdom. There will be famines and earthquakes in various places. All these are the beginning of birth pains.

Some may think that the end of age is near because world wars did happen and the wars today are really heavy and the area involved is also great compared to those in the past: these are the reflection of the Bible saying that kingdoms rose against kingdoms and nations against nations, famines, pestilences, and earthquakes in various places. I will not object. However, some may ask that since the history of human, wars indeed were common; kingdoms always rose against kingdoms and nations against nations; there had been always famines, pestilences, and earthquakes in various places. How can we say that nowadays, in the twentieth century, is near the end of age exactly as Jesus meant?

If we concentrate on the meaning of the word **"hear"** in that sentence, we may have some ideals of what Jesus said. It is true that there were always wars and kingdom rose against kingdom and nation against nation, as well as famines, pestilences, and earthquakes in various places. However, one could hardly get news even of a war right next to him. The communication before the computer era was actually poor. The transmission of information had unacceptable time lag. After the intervention of computer and world-wide-web, transmission of information can reach anywhere within seconds. That is why information technology (IT) is also called information superhighway. In this twentieth century, you cannot deny that you must "**hear**" news everyday through TVs, newspapers, telephones, mobiles, Internet and E-mails. You can easily read the news by seeing the newspaper held by a person next to you. You do not need to buy it. It occurs inside the underground railway everyday. Although wars, famines, pestilences, and earthquakes in various places have been always happening since there was human, only in this century does one begin to "**hear**" it.

It is therefore one of the supportive evidences that the end of age is near. Do you believe it ?

References:

1. Cohen, N.L., Waltzman, S.B., Fisher, S.G., for The Department of Veterans Affairs Cochlear Implant S1tudy Group. "A Prospective, Randomized Study of Cochlear Implants." *New Eng J Med* 1993; 328 (4) : 233–237.
2. Seidman, M.D., Ahmad, N., Bai, U., "Molecular mechanisms of age-related hearing loss." *Ageing Res Rev.* 2002 Jun.1(3):331–43.

Chapter 23

The Law Concerning Our Teeth (Dentistry)

A Common Chronic Disease

Do you know what the most common chronic disease of children aged five to seventeen is? Is it asthma or child abuse?

No, it is dental caries (tooth decay) and it is five times more common than asthma (59% versus 11%). Of course, adults have untreated dental caries, too; it is about 27% of those thirty-five to forty-four years old and 30% of those sixty-five years and older [2]. Enamel of our teeth in fact is the hardest part of our body but it can still decay by the acid production of bacteria in our oral cavity. It may be difficult and impractical to prevent children from candy. Therefore to control dental caries effectively, we have to teach our children to clean their teeth after eating. For adults, the most effective way is to stop smoking.

The Functions Of Our Teeth

The main functions of the teeth are of course for chewing and to assist eating. It is also play some roles in producing accurate speech sounds. Apart from these, the teeth are also of paramount importance in our social life. They give us confident appearance. Old people may like to have denture for improving their chewing ability and appearance. Even a young girl of age six would be reluctant to smile if she lost her milk tooth in front of her mouth. We always underestimate the importance of having good teeth to one's social life.

A Tooth For A Tooth

In the Old Testament, an eye for an eye and a tooth for a tooth is a law (Matthew 5:38). It aimed at limiting the revenge by a clear statement. However, is it really clear enough to implement in our real life? It may be easily understood that when someone hit my left eye leading to blindness, his left eye should be sacrificed in order to compensate for my loss. We have only two eyes and it may be easy for us to calculate. Do you know how many teeth an adult has? Twenty-eight or thirty-two?

In childhood, there are twenty deciduous teeth (milk teeth) and the replacement of thirty-two permanent teeth usually completed by the age of eighteen. However, some may have between twenty-eight to thirty-two teeth as the third molars (wisdom teeth) impacted within the gum [1]. For an adult, he will have four medial incisors, four lateral incisors, four canines, four first premolars, four second premolars, four first molars, four second molars and four wisdom teeth.

The Law Concerning Our Teeth (Dentistry)

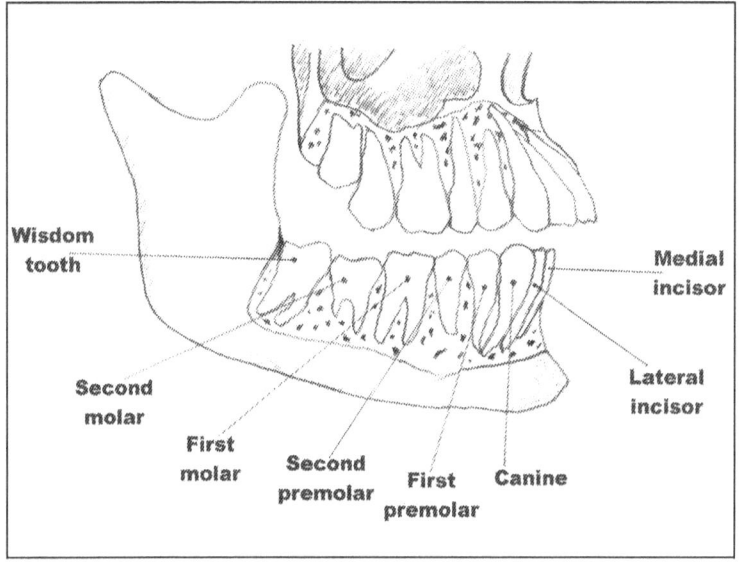

Figure 23.1 The position of teeth

It may be well understood that if someone hit my mouth leading to a lost of the left upper medial incisor, the same tooth of that person therefore should be sacrificed in order to compensate my loss. If someone breaks my wisdom tooth but I find that he has no wisdom tooth (because of impaction), how can he compensate for my loss? Or if he had already compensated the tooth for another person before hitting me, how can I ask for that revenge? The law therefore may not be enough for my case. In fact, is our law today versatile for us in order to live in a fair community? How do we develop a perfect law in order to protect everyone's right without any loss?

The Law Of Compensation

In Matthew 5: 1–2, 38–48

Now when he saw the crowds, he went up on a

mountainside and sat down. His disciples came to him, and he began to teach them saying: "You have heard that it was said, 'An eye for eye, and **tooth for tooth**.' But I tell you, Do not resist an evil person. If someone strikes you on the right cheek, turn to him the other also. And if someone wants to sue you and take your tunic, let him have your cloak as well. If someone forces you to go one mile, go with him two miles. Give to the one who asks you, and do not turn away from the one who wants to borrow from you.

"You have heard that it was said, 'Love your neighbor and hate your enemy.' But I tell you: Love your enemies and pray for those who persecute you, that you may be sons of your Father in heaven. He causes his sun to rise on the evil and the good, and sends rain on the righteous and the unrighteous. If you love those who love you, what reward will you get? Are not even the tax collectors doing that? And if you greet only your brothers, what are you doing more than others? Do not even pagans do that? Be perfect, therefore, as your heavenly Father is perfect."

The teaching by Jesus above is strange. If someone slaps our right cheek, it may be fine for us not to revenge by slapping back his right cheek. It may be good to stop here. But why should we have to turn to the other side for him to slap another? If someone wants to sue us and takes our tunic, it is so generous that we do not ask him back for his tunic and sue him back. But why should we even give him our cloak? If someone compels us to walk one mile for him, we will be very nice to do it without asking back for the mile. But why should we walk another mile extra? Obviously, the one slaps our cheek, sues us with our tunic and compels us to walk one mile is not our friend. Why should we need to do that extra for our enemy?

The Law Concerning Our Teeth (Dentistry)

Obviously, it is not a law as it cannot protect the victim and it is simply not fair. The result of doing such thing is **suffering**. Very likely, you will be slapped again, sued successfully and exhausted for the extra mile. Therefore what is this teaching?

It is not a law. It is love. Foolish people like me always can hardly understand it. It teaches us how to suffer. The translation of 1 Corinthians 13 in New King James Version is "Love **suffers** long." In New International Version is "Love is patient." Indeed, how patient is considered to be patient enough? For someone slapping me, how patient should I be in order to be considered patient enough? Patient until suffering? How many times should I forgive my brothers? How many times should I suffer from the one who slaps me?

What Is Love

Every Christian knows where to find the definition of love in the Bible. It is inside 1 Corinthians 13. But what does it mean?

Paul said, "Though I speak with the tongues of men and of angels, but have not love, I have become as sounding brass or a clanging cymbal."

"Though I have the gift of prophecy, and understand all mysteries and all knowledge, but have not love, I am nothing." Can a man have all knowledge and understand all mysteries? Wow, he must be something if he really can. However, Paul said that man could still be nothing. Well, it seems to be strange.

Paul continued to say, "Though I have all faith, so that I could remove mountains, but have not love, I am nothing." Well, it is even strange. A faith that can move not just one mountain but many mountains should be highly appreciated by Jesus. I can quote thousands of verses from the Bible that

Jesus would love that man with all faith. So, how could Paul say that he could still be nothing? Was Paul too old to think about this logic? How could this be?

Paul continued to say, "And though I bestow all my goods to feed the poor, and though I give my body to be burned, but have not love, it profits me nothing." Now Paul must be mad. How could a man give out all he has and even his body without love and be nothing. He was really mad. No one could believe that. How could this be?

Paul then explained what is the real meaning of love. He said, "Love suffers long . . ." (New King James Version)

Yes . . . Love suffers long.

After hearing just the first sentence, I knew that I was wrong. I kneeled down inevitably and felt that I was foolish and I knew nothing. I am nothing, too. For love is measured in terms of **time**.

Do you know why a man giving out all he has to the poor could still be without love?

I have seen a female patient recently. She was thirty-eight years old and was married for many years. She and her husband did not want any children and she has taken oral or injection contraceptive method for many years. As she was approaching forty, her obstetrician advised her to change to other contraceptive methods such as barrier method since the side effects of pills may outweigh the benefits. She asked the obstetrician to do the operation for her contraception but many times she was rejected. Do you know why? Why was the obstetrician reluctant to operate on her so that she could never be pregnant anymore?

It is simply because we always change. We always do things because of impulse. We thought we would not but actually we always change. We always change our mind, our attitude, our behavior and our mood. It may be even more common for women influenced by fluctuations of hormones in their climacteric period. It did happen that patients who underwent irreversible sterilization operation wanted to get pregnant again and finally sued the doctors. She might not be wrong to change her mind as everything around her was changing, too. Perhaps her husband was dying with cancer and she wanted a baby from her husband, or she just felt lonely and wanted a baby. We all change. We always think that we would not have done something but indeed we did it. We did it and regretted and we do it again. The things we do may be just an impulsive action. It may be influenced by our surrounding people, peer, social environment, economic status, mood, and internal hormones.

Can a man giving out all he has or even his body still be without love?

Yes, he can. The underlying reasons for him to do that action can be many. Love is only one of them. It may be due to other things such as impulse, mood, hormones, etc. I have a friend who is a surgeon. I can still remember some years ago when he spent nearly all his money in just a night because the girl he loved rejected him. He asked me to accompany him and we dined out in a very expensive restaurant. He gave great tips to the waiters, and to the poor. It was not because he loved the waiters or the poor. It was because he felt rejected and he wanted to release. In fact, many people like to spend money to release their sadness when they are unhappy. Fortunately, the girl who rejected him is his wife now. He does not spend money like that because he loves money now.

So, again, what is love?

Paul told us that love suffers long. That means love is measured in terms of time, like the love of God. He loved you and me since our birth and till we die. That love never changes even if we sinned and regretted so many times. Every time we repent, his love to us is the same. It will not decrease because we have sinned for so many times. That love never fails. He loves us from His creation to the end of age. He persists even though we hurt Him. He suffers the longest.

Now this is love. This love cannot be understood by others. It persists, never changes and fails. There is suffering inside.

We don't know love

Every Valentine's day, one question must be asked in the radio program? Do you know what this is? This is: "What will you do to your boyfriend or girlfriend in Valentine's Day in order to show that you love him or her?"

The answers are nearly the same every year without creativity. I do not know why we lack creativity nowadays. For example, buy her these kinds of flowers, those kinds of presents, bring her to someplace for a surprise or a romantic night, prepare her some expensive or handmade products, etc. All is "doing this and doing that" in order to make her feel his love.

Is it really love? What does Paul tell us about love?

In 1 Corinthians 13, Paul told us that love does not envy, does not parade itself, is not puffed up, does not behave rudely, does not seek its own, is not provoked, thinks no evil; does not rejoice in iniquity, but rejoices in the truth, bear all things, believes all things, hopes all things, endures all things.

Love is not "doing this and doing that." Love is "not doing this and not doing that," **not** envy; **not** parade itself, **not** puffed up; **not** behave rudely, **not** seek its own, **not** provoked, thinks **no** evil; **not** rejoice in iniquity. There is no use in buying her an expensive present but still envy on her. There is no use in giving her a surprise when you behave rudely after her surprise. There is no use in preparing her a romantic night but you think all evil. There is no use giving her a handmade product if you get provoked and angry easily. We thought we showed our love by doing something but, in fact, we did not. We are sinners. Only can we prevent ourselves from doing something so that we may know love. Love is "not doing this and not doing that." We would never know what love is if it had not been written in the Bible.

Next time, when this question is asked again in the radio program, dial up to the host and tell him about this.

References:

1. Liebgott, B. *The anatomical basis of dentistry.* (Philadelphia: WB Saunders Co.) 1982.
2. Centers for Disease Control and Prevention (CDC). "Preventing Chronic Diseases: Investing Wisely in Health. Preventing Dental Caries" [http://www.cdc.gov/OralHealth/factsheets/dental_caries.htm –assessed on 3rd December 2002]

Chapter 24

X-rays and the Judgment of Jesus (Radiology)

When Was X-rays Discover

Wilhelm Konrad Roentgen, a German physicist, discovered X-rays as a powerful diagnostic tool on 1895 when he passed electricity through vacuum tubes with barium platinocyanide in his experiment. Different tissues can be "seen" under this new technique and it was then used immediately in hospitals to diagnose fractures, bone diseases and foreign bodies. Roentgen was awarded a Nobel Prize in 1901 because of this important breakthrough in the modern medicine [3].

How Many Medical Imaging Techniques To "See" A Person Nowadays

There are at least seven:

1. X-rays with or without other radioactive substances
2. Ultrasound
3. Radioactive Imaging
4. Computed Tomography (CT)

5. Positron Emission Tomography (PET)
6. Single Photon Emission Computed Tomography (SPECT)
7. Magnetic Resonance Imaging (MRI)

Traditionally, structural imaging techniques such as X-rays, CT, MRI and ultrasound have been considered versatile in the diagnosis of diseases. One can see the cross-sections of a human in different planes: transverse cut, longitudinal cut, etc. MRI is no doubted to be the most powerful tool among all imaging techniques in terms of clarity. Although it is now inferior to CT in chest and abdomen imaging, MRI will surely catch up quickly. In fact, the imaging techniques have been evolving since these three to four decades [1]; Computed Tomography (CT) was introduced in 1972 [2], PET in 1975 [4], SPECT in 1976 [5] and MRI in 1980.

Can We Read People's Minds By Imaging Techniques

Previously we thought that it was impossible to read people's minds, but now we have to change.

In Matthew 5: 27–30 (Adultery)

Jesus said, "You have heard that it was said, 'Do not commit adultery.' But I tell you that anyone who **looks** at a woman lustfully has already committed adultery with her in his heart. If your right eye causes you to sin, gouge it out and throw it away. It is better for you to lose one part of your body than for your whole body to be thrown into hell. And if your right hand causes you to sin, cut it off and throw it away. It is better for you to lose one part of your body than for your whole body to go into hell."

In Matthew 5: 27–30, Jesus commended his disciples not to sin from his heart. Whoever looks at a girl lustfully commits adultery. Some may ask that how can others know what one thinks when he is looking at a girl? How do we know what he thinks in his mind? Or how can others know whether one wants to kill another if there is no evidence of plan or action? We may think that only God can 'see' our minds. Other people must not.

Today, we may think about the above questions again and revise our answers after the exploding evolution of functional imaging. The world indeed has changed.

What Is Functional Imaging

Functional imaging is the technique used to "see" the function of the human body by imaging. These new techniques include PET, SPECT, and functional MRI. PET and SPECT can detect different metabolism in human organs and reflect with different colors and signals [6, 7]. For example, the signals of cancer cells and normal cells are different because of their different glucose transport. The resolutions however are not very good. Functional MRI is different; the structural image produced is clear and functional activities of some organs, say brain, can be depicted simultaneously. For instance, the visual part of the brain will be signaled in a different color when one's vision is simulated or the finger part of the brain is colored when one is moving his fingers. The reason behind this is the detection of increasing blood flow and oxygen or tiny movements of water particles (protons) over a few microns [1 micron = 0.001 mm] [6].

To See People's Minds

By these advancing techniques of imaging, our thoughts

indeed can be "seen" possibly in the near future. If a man looks at a woman with indecent thoughts, recent functional imaging may detect it. First of all, the visual part of the brain will increase signaling as blood flow increases. The area of brain associated with genital organ of that man will also increase in blood flow and oxygen that may be depicted by functional imaging. We may conclude that what he sees is related to his increase sexual desire.

When we smile, one set of muscles contracts. And when we are angry, another set of muscles contracts (e.g., our jaw muscles clench). The areas of brain controlling these muscles will increase in blood flow and imaging can detect these changes in signals. Future advancing imaging may detect these tiny increase blood and water flow although the person tries to hide this manifestation by not contracting these facial muscles. He cannot hide his thoughts in his brain. By observing the functional imaging, we therefore can know that what he sees makes him angry or happy.

In the future, it may also be used in National Security Agency to detect lies from a spy. For example, we may put him in functional MRI and talk to him with some true statements. Then we observe his body scans with different signal combination. After that, we talk to him with some false statements and observing his body scans again. Finally, we test him with a statement we do not know whether it is true or false. We may then observe the scan result to see whether it is like those scans from true statements or those from false statements. We may therefore know that it is a lie or not even the spy may be keeping silent all along.

Therefore it is not completely impossible to see people's minds in the future. And we may be wrong if we think that only God can 'see' our minds.

The Judgment Of Jesus

In Matthew 5: 21–26, (Murder)

"You have heard that it was said to the people long ago, 'Do not murder, and anyone who murders will be subject to judgment.' But I tell you that anyone who is angry with his brother will be subject to judgment. Again, anyone who says to his brother, 'Raca,' is answerable to the Sanhedrin. But anyone who says, 'You fool!' will be in danger of the fire of hell.

"Therefore, if you are offering your gift at the altar and there remember that your brother has something against you, leave your gift there in front of the altar. First go and be reconciled to your brother; then come and offer your gift.

"Settle matters quickly with your adversary who is taking you to court. Do it while you are still with him on the way, or he may hand you over to the judge, and the judge may hand you over to the officer, and you may be thrown into prison. I tell you the truth, you will not get out until you have paid the last penny."

References:

1. Gray, JE, Orton, CG. *Medical Physics: Some Recollections in Diagnostic X-ray Imaging and Therapeutic Radiology*, 2000; 217 (3): 619–625.
2. Hounsfield, GH. Computerized transverse axial scanning (tomography). I. Description of the system. Br J Radiol 1973; 68: 166–172.
3. Margotta R. "X-rays and other means of diagnosis." In: *The Hamlyn History of Medicine*. (London: Reed International Books Ltd, 1996), pp. 170–7.

4. Ter-Pogossian MM, Phelps ME, Hoffman EJ, Mullani NA. "A positron-emission transaxial tomography for nuclear imaging (PETT)." *Radiology*, 1975; 114:89–98.
5. Society of Nuclear Medicine. *The history of nuclear medicine*. Available at: www.snm.org/nuclear/history.html
6. Hawnaur, J. "Clinical review: Recent advances Diagnostic radiology." *BMJ* 1999; 319: 168–71.
7. Jagust, W, Thisted, R, Devous, MD, Van Heertum, R, Mayberg, H, Jobst, K, Smith, AD and Borys, N. "SPECT perfusion imaging in the diagnosis of Alzheimer's disease: A clinical-pathologic study." *Neurology* 2001; 56: 950–956.

Chapter 25

Similarity between Sin and Cancer (Oncology)

What Is Oncology

Oncology is the study of cancers and their prevention, diagnosis and management, including chemotherapy (killing cancer with drugs), radiotherapy (killing cancer with irradiation), palliative (non-curing, relieving) treatment and pain control in a holistic approach. New treatments such as gene therapy, immunotherapy and some new drugs now appear and may add some benefits in selected patients [1]. Gene therapy is the idea of introducing normal genes into the cells of patients who has defective genes. Immunotherapy tries to modify the tumor cells so that the immune system of the patient can identify and kill them effectively. However, these new treatment modalities are only in the experimental stage.

What Are The Causes Of Cancer

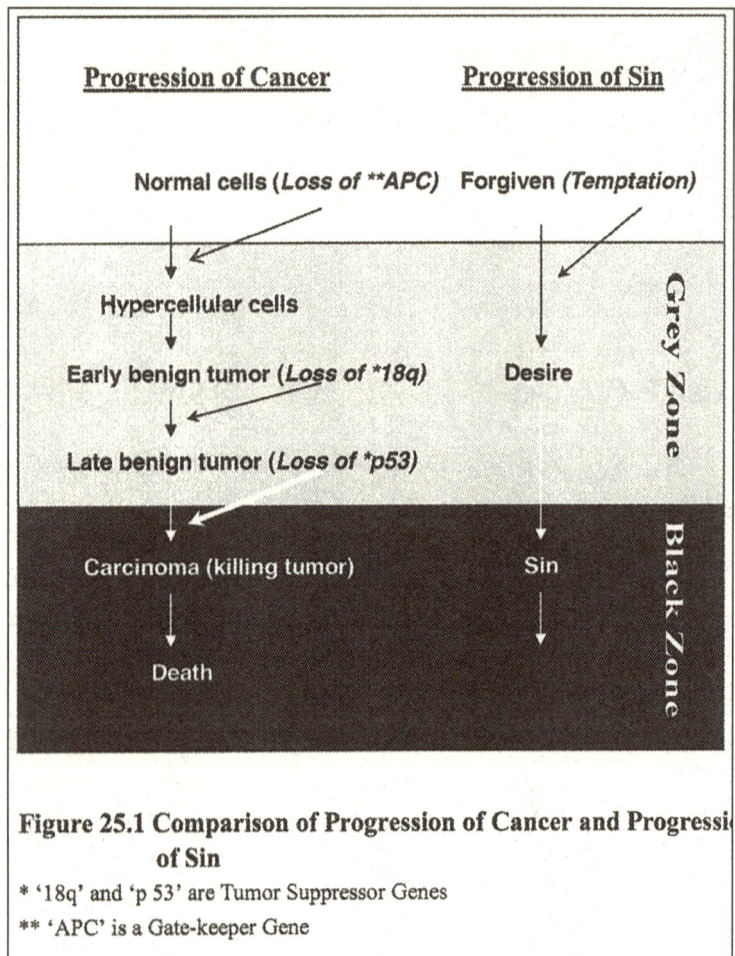

Figure 25.1 Comparison of Progression of Cancer and Progression of Sin

* '18q' and 'p 53' are Tumor Suppressor Genes
** 'APC' is a Gate-keeper Gene

It was suggested that the progression of cancer is a multi-step process. Mutation (sudden change) of genes may occur at different sites to initiate the cancer progress. It follows by genetic changes to produce the intermediate non-killing tumor and final killing cancer [2]. There may be at least an initiative and a promoting process. Say for example in colon cancer, the first step may include the loss of the "gatekeeper" gene that leads to the initiation of the cancer process [3]. The intermediate non-killing tumors are produced after some other genetic modifications. It is illustrated as the Grey Zone in Figure. 25.1. Continued loss of some tumor-suppressor genes leads to the ultimate progression of the final killing cancer [4]. This promotion process is illustrated as the Black Zone in Figure 25.1.

What Are The Causes Of Sin

Most of the times, it is difficult to define which behavior or action is sinful. Unlawful is not equivalent to sinful. Gambling, smoking and attending sexual workers are legal in many countries but are they absolutely free of sinful nature? To be more difficult: how about telling lies or giving false hope to comfort a dying patient? There is no absolute and universal definition of sinful behavior for all cultures. Perhaps most of these are just like the progression of cancer.

When we are forgiven by the Lord through the blood of Jesus, we are totally clean and holy. We are in the white area as illustrated in Figure 25.1. However, temptations are all around to move our will and decision to follow Jesus. In fact, the temptations are all "suggestions" from Satan. It cannot change our mind unless we make a deal with its suggestion. These temptations just like the environmental hazards such as carcinogenic food, harmful radiation from the earth and the universe. They want us to 'mutate' and start the progress to 'cancer'. Some suggestions may not immediately lead to sin but evil desires. For example: Just a lie to comfort a poor patient, is not a problem, at least to him. Just not giving to the poor is all right, maybe I can just pray for them more in order to compensate it. Gambling just once as it is the company's annual activity.

In James 1: 14–15

But each one is tempted when, by his own evil desire, he is dragged away and enticed. Then, after desire has conceived, it gives birth to sin; and sin, when it is full grown, gives birth to death.

Point Of No Return

When we make a deal with the suggestion from Satan, we are at least in the Grey Zone. We have already started the progress to 'cancer'. We may not notice it but God will remind us as He is faithful. Evil desires will accumulate and progress, like the promotion phase in the development of cancer. Until you reach a point to enter the Black Zone, you discover that there is no return. Can one say that if I know what or where is the point of no return, then I can still control myself and not enter it and enjoy in my evil desires without death. However, in the progress to sin and death, the point of no return is usually difficult to notice. When we notice it, sometimes it is too late. Like Judas who betrayed Jesus, he could not repent although he felt guilty later. In the beginning, he just stole money but finally he killed his master indirectly. In fact, the point of no return in the progression of cancer or the progression of sin may not be actually a "point." It may be not necessarily a fixed position and can be different from person to person.

Can patients suffering from benign colon tumor be reassured that it will never progress to cancer in the rest of his life? How about if his life span can increase fifty or one hundred years? Are all benign tumors absolutely benign if one's life span is increased? In fact, if the time is really long enough, say hundreds of years, all benign colon tumors are able to progress to cancer. This is similar to that of the progression of evil desire. If one could live forever, all evil desire will become sin no matter how slow it progresses. That is why God must make us clean without even a trace of evil desire in His eternal kingdom.

In the management of cancer, it is always true that prevention is better than treatment. It is more effective, inexpensive, and decreases sufferings. It may also be true to deal with the progression of sin. Tackle the evil desires as early as possible in Lord Jesus as suggested by James. It is more effective, costs less (you lose little), and much comfortable.

References:

1. Tattersall, MHN, Thomas, H. "Clinical review: Recent advances Oncology" *BMJ* 1999; 318: 445–8.
2. Kinzler, KW, Vogelstein, B. "Multi-step carcinogenesis: Lessons from hereditary colorectal cancer." *Cell* 1996; 87: 159.
3. Kinzler, KW, Vogelstein, B. "Gatekeeper and caretakers." *Nature* 1997; 386: 761.
4. Cotran, RS, Kumar, V, Collins, T. "Neoplasia." In: Robbins *Pathologic Basis of Disease*, 6th eds. (Philadelphia: WB Saunders Co, 1999), pp. 260–328.

Chapter 26

Did Jesus Have Anxiety? (Psychiatry)

Living in a busy world, we all have been experiencing anxiety. If you have a job, you will probably be stressed everyday. If you do not have a job, you will probably have more stress for finding one. In fact, a baby in his mother's womb starts to face stress, physical stress like pressure of the womb and chemical stress like hypoxia (inadequate oxygen). Mentally retarded people do have stress, too. They may cry when they feel stressful or uncomfortable. No one therefore is immunized to stress.

What Is Anxiety

We all have anxiety and peace inside us is always not enough.

Anxiety is somewhat different from anxiety disorder. Psychiatrists tend to agree that anxiety disorder may need some reliable and valid criteria. Two most influential classifications applied nowadays are the Diagnostic and Statistical Manual of mental disorders, 4th edition (DSM IV) [1] and International statistical Classification of Diseases and related health problems, 10th revision (ICD 10) [2]. They agree that to classify an anxiety disorder, symptoms like trembling, feeling shaky, aching in the back and shoulders, tension headaches, chest tightness, restlessness, exaggerated startle, irritability, insomnia, fatigue, dry mouth, **sweating**, urinary frequency, trouble swallowing, nausea, and diarrhea may need to be present for some time and affect our daily and social living. The worries are also more pervasive and difficult to control than normal worries [3]. We may not have anxiety disorder but we must surely have worries.

Did Jesus Have Anxiety

It is no doubt that Jesus had no sin. But did he have weakness? If yes, what was his weakness?

In Luke 22: 39–44, (Jesus Prays on the Mount of Olives)

Jesus went out as usual to the Mount of Olives ... He withdrew about a stone's throw beyond them, knelt down and prayed, "Father, if you are willing, take this cup from me; yet not my will, but yours be done." An angel from heaven appeared to him and strengthened him. And being in anguish, he prayed more earnestly, and his **sweat** was like drops of blood falling to the ground.

I believe that Jesus had weakness during the time in human history otherwise Satan's temptation would become meaningless. So what was his weakness?

Perhaps we can find some evidence from the temptations from Satan.

In Matthew 4:3

The tempter came to him and said, "**If you are the Son of God**, tell these stones to become bread."

Did Jesus Have Anxiety? (Psychiatry)

In Matthew 4:6

"**If you are the Son of God**," he said, "throw yourself down. For it is written: 'He will command his angels concerning you, and they will lift you up in their hands, so that you will not strike your foot against a stone.'"

Satan was very clever. In his temptations, which words were repeated frequently? Yes, it is: "**If you are the Son of God . . .**"
Why did the chief of all evil spirits, Satan, challenge Jesus with this: How to prove the identity "a Son of God"?
Some people may think that to prove yourself as son of God, you should at least do some extraordinary events that humans cannot do. Jesus, already reached his thirty, had no experience in even one single miracle. So the question that had to be asked of Jesus was: "Who told you that you are the son of God?" Okay, if you are really a son of God, do a miracle before me to verify that." It was in fact a sensible request for Jesus announcement.
After the temptation in the beginning of the salvation, did Satan really leave Jesus alone? It seemed not. The chief of all evil spirits, Satan, did appear again when Jesus was thirsty in the end of his salvation.

Two robbers were crucified with him, one on his right and one on his left. Those who passed by hurled insults at him, shaking their heads and saying, "You who are going to destroy the temple and build it in three days, save yourself! Come down from the cross, if you are the Son of God!" (Matthew 27: 38–40)

The words appeared again when Jesus was thirty: "**If you are the Son of God . . .**"

In fact, these words appeared once when he was hungry. Now the last temptation came when he was thirsty. "Come down. Why suffer? I believe that You are the Son of God now. Come down first." The first temptation in the wild when Jesus was hungry was indeed rude and full of challenge. But the last temptation on the cross when he was thirsty was really full of "sympathy." "Come down, I believe you. The son of God should not need to suffer here. Come down."

We understand here that the weakness or the anxiety behind Jesus might be related to his assurance of the identity as "a Son of God."

If this is really a source of anxiety in Jesus, how did God Himself solve this problem? Exempt Jesus from those temptations? It seemed not. Perhaps we might find some evidence from the experiences when Jesus met the Father.

In Luke 3; 21–22, (The Baptism)

When all the people were being baptized, Jesus was baptized, too. And as he was praying, heaven was opened and the Holy Spirit descended on him in bodily form like a dove. And a voice came from heaven: "**You are my Son**, whom I love; with you I am well pleased."

In Matthew 17:1–5, (The Transfiguration)

After six days, Jesus took with him Peter, James and John, the brother of James, and led them up a high mountain by themselves. There he was transfigured before them. His face shone like the sun, and his clothes became as white as the light . . . a bright cloud enveloped them, and a voice from the cloud said, "**This is my Son**, whom I love; with him I am well pleased. Listen to him!"

God seemed to ease the possible anxiety behind Jesus by repeated reassurance. "This is my beloved Son . . ." These words were surely spoken for the sake of Jesus and the people around him. For every adopted child, the most common problem arising inside may be his own identity. "Who am I?", "Am I unwanted?", "Did I do something wrong so that my birth parents forsook me?" [4]

Jesus was somewhat like an "adopted" child growing in the family of Joseph and Mary. The possible weakness or anxiety arising from identity confusion might affect him as he was also a human on earth. He did have feelings and emotions. He wept (John 11: 35), he got angry (Matthew 21: 12–13), he moved with compassion (Mark 1: 41), he felt hungry (Matthew 4: 2).

Perhaps the most effective way to alleviate this kind of identity confusion is reassurance, especially coming from the Father.

Do Christians have a more flattened road in their life? Are they all immunized to anxiety? Of course, the answer is no. Just like Jesus, all Christians have their difficulties in life and their roads are not flattened comparing others, sometimes it is harder. It seems that God does not promise to take away all difficulties in Christian's life. However, just like Jesus, God has promised us peace — a peace that cannot be taken away.

Peace I leave with you; my peace I give you. I do not give to you as the world gives. Do not let your hearts be troubled and do not be afraid. (John 14: 27)

Although the storms outside are heavy, it is peaceful inside.

"The Lord will fight for you, and you shall hold your peace." (Exodus 14: 14 [New King James Version])

References:

1. American Psychiatric Association: *Diagnostic and Statistical Manual of Mental Disorders*, 4th ed. (Washington, DC: American Psychiatric Association, 1994).
2. World Health Organization. *International statistical classification of diseases and related health problems*, 10th revision. (Geneva: WHO, 1992).
3. Spiegel, DA, Barlow, DH. "Generalized anxiety disorders." In: Michael G. Gelder, Juan J. López-Ibor Jr, Nancy C. Andreasen. *New Oxford Textbook of Psychiatry*, 1st ed. (New York: Oxford University Press, 2000).
4. Nickman, SL. "Adoption." In: Harold I. Kaplan, M.D, Benjamin J. Sadock, M.D and Virginia A. Sadock, M.D. *Kaplan & Sadock's Comprehensive Textbook of Psychiatry*, 7th ed. (USA: Lippincott Williams & Wilkins, 2000).

At last . . .

Writing a book, in fact, is not easy. It is not only the time you have to sacrifice but also things you do not expect, such as your heart and soul.

It is not easy when you face every difficulty in the journey of writing, like the journey of our life. There were excitations and depressions. For someone (like me) who lacks the image of a father, it may be especially hard to overcome those difficulties. The image of a father in a child's heart is the power to protect, the strength to overcome and the comfort to depress. We can never avoid difficulties and depressions in our life. In cities where the divorce rates are notoriously high, it is even difficult to find enough comfort, strength and power. How can we deal with those hard times?

Jesus, once a human on the earth, lacked the image of a father as well. Some people believe that Joseph, father of Jesus, was dead when he was young. I also have the same belief. In a male-dominant society like old Jerusalem, people were usually named "the son of someone (name of his father)." Jesus, however, was always named the son of Mary but not the son of Joseph. It might be the fact that he was born by Mary alone. When Jesus was crucified, he asked John to look after his mother but not father. Obviously, Joseph was not there when Jesus was being hung.

How can Jesus overcome so much difficulties in his daily life when most of the times powerful people wanted to kill him? For not so many times had he been reassured by God to be His beloved son (maybe many times privately).

Where can we get our strength when there is sorrow?

Where can we find a father again?

Father, how a beautiful name it can be, how important his love to us and what will happen if we do not have one.

In John 1: 12–13

Yet to all who received him, to those who believed in his name, he gave the right to become **children of God** — children born not of natural descent, nor of human decision or a husband's will, but born of God.

Finally, I hope this book can help people who were, who are or who will be, in trouble. I also hope that this book can be edited to keep in touch with our fast developing medical science. Shall I invite you here again to write, if possible, a series of music in Bible, economics in Bible, architecture in Bible, etc?

May the Most High, Almighty God bless us until Jesus returns.

Amen.

Author's Biography

John WK Yeung is a Christian and was baptized in 1994. He received his Bachelor of Medicine and Bachelor of Surgery (MBBS) from Hong Kong University in 1996. He later graduated from Chinese University of Hong Kong in 2002 with a Master of Sciences in Epidemiology and Biostatistics (MSc). He lives with his wife who is a nurse and a paper clay craftsman. The author believes the knowledge today is compatible with the holy Bible.

For details, please visit: www.MedicineInBible.com

Book Summary

What was the possible cause of Jesus' death?
Were the Ten Plagues related to microorganism infection?
Did Adam have one rib less than Eve?
Why did King David need a young girl to treat his coldness when he was old?
Did Jesus have anxiety?
Why were the hairs of Absalom so heavy?
What was the purpose of sour wine in crucifixion?
How could Jesus become bright during the transfiguration?
How did circumcision reveal the intelligence of God?
Can we "hear" the End of Age?
and more . . .

The author wants to share his opinion with you in this book.

www.ingramcontent.com/pod-product-compliance
Lightning Source LLC
Chambersburg PA
CBHW030935180526
45163CB00002B/576